Psychiatric and Cognitive Disorders in Parkinson's Disease

Emotional and cognitive disorders are common in Parkinson's disease, but are frequently overlooked or undertreated. This book provides a comprehensive account of these aspects of Parkinson's disease, based on the neurologic and psychiatric assessment of hundreds of patients by the authors. It also offers a thorough survey of the published literature on the topic.

Readers will find a complete and helpful overview of the clinical features and treatment of Parkinson's disease, followed by discussion of associated depressive disorders, anxiety, phobias, apathy, hallucinations, delusions and sleep disorders. Specific cognitive deficits are also discussed, and the mechanisms for these disorders explored. In addition, the book addresses the psychiatric and cognitive side-effects of antiparkinsonian medications and new surgical treatments.

Offering sufficient scientific detail for the specialist in neurology and psychiatry, the clear practical guidelines, case studies and rating scales will meet the needs of all clinicians working with Parkinson's disease patients.

Sergio E. Starkstein was Assistant Professor of Psychiatry at Johns Hopkins University, and is now head of the Dementia Clinic at the La Sagrada Familia Clinic, and Director of the Buenos Aires Neuropsychiatric Center.

Marcelo Merello was a Research Fellow at the National Hospital for Neurology and Neurosurgery in London, and is now head of the Movement Disorders Section (FLENI) in Buenos Aires.

Psychiatric
and **Cognitive Disorders**
in **Parkinson's Disease**

Sergio E. Starkstein
La Sagrada Familia Clinic and Buenos Aires Neuropsychiatric Center
Buenos Aires, Argentina

Marcelo Merello
Raúl Carrea Institute of Neurological Research-FLENI
Buenos Aires, Argentina

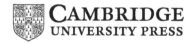
CAMBRIDGE
UNIVERSITY PRESS

CAMBRIDGE UNIVERSITY PRESS
Cambridge, New York, Melbourne, Madrid, Cape Town, Singapore, São Paulo

Cambridge University Press
The Edinburgh Building, Cambridge CB2 8RU, UK

Published in the United States of America by Cambridge University Press, New York

www.cambridge.org
Information on this title: www.cambridge.org/9780521663052

First published 2002
This digitally printed version 2007

A catalogue record for this publication is available from the British Library

Library of Congress Cataloguing in Publication data

Starkstein, Sergio E.
Psychiatric and cognitive disorders in Parkinson's disease / Sergio E. Starkstein,
Marcelo J. Merello.
    p. cm.
Includes bibliographical references and index.
ISBN 0 521 66305 9
1. Parkinson's disease – Patients – Mental health. 2. Psychological manifestations of
general diseases. I. Merello, Marcelo J., 1961– II. Title.
[DNLM: 1. Parkinson Disease – psychology. 2. Mental Disorders. WL 359 S795p 2002]
RC382.S72 2002
6161.8'33'0019–dc21 2001043116

ISBN 978-0-521-66305-2 hardback
ISBN 978-0-521-66398-4 paperback

Every effort has been made in preparing this book to provide accurate and up-to-date information which
is in accord with accepted standards and practice at the time of publication. Nevertheless, the authors,
editors and publisher can make no warranties that the information contained herein is totally free from error,
not least because standards are constantly changing through research and regulation. The authors, editors
and publisher therefore disclaim all liability for direct or consequential damages resulting from the use of
material contained in this book. Readers are strongly advised to pay careful attention to information provided
by the manufacturer of any drugs or equipment that they plan to use.

For our beloved wives, Corina and Alicia

Contents

Preface

As part of our clinical and research activities in neurology and psychiatry, we had the chance to examine hundreds of patients with Parkinson's disease (PD). The Movement Disorders Unit kept us abreast of the new developments in the management of the clinical complications of PD, and made us aware of the emotional, behavioral, and cognitive complications of the disease. These problems have been specifically studied at the Departments of Neuropsychiatry of our Institutes, where we carry out most of our clinical and research activities in the interface between neurology and psychiatry.

Whereas emotional problems such as depression and anxiety are very prevalent in PD, they are rarely diagnosed and treated. One of the reasons for the low awareness of mood problems in PD is that some of the key symptoms of depression, such as psychomotor retardation, lack of energy, loss of libido, insomnia, and low energy, are also frequently found among PD patients. There may also be a tendency to "expect" PD patients to be somewhat depressed based on their physical limitations, and to consider depressed mood as an "understandable" consequence of the illness. On the other hand, behavioral problems such as delusions and hallucinations dramatically affect both patients' and caregivers' lives, and treatment is readily obtained. Cognitive disorders slowly develop in a high proportion of PD patients, and the familial and financial impact of this complication is comparable to that in other dementias.

Thus, it is frequently the case that a PD patient with moderate or severe disease is burdened by a variety of clinical problems, such as a progressive depressive mood, worries about their motor problems, loss of self-confidence, and avoidance of social situations where their motor difficulties may become manifest. Tremor and akinesia tend to increase dramatically in social situations, leading to episodes of "freezing." Patients are usually well aware of these potential complications, and tend to avoid social contact by staying at home. With the progression of the illness, many PD patients develop cognitive deficits that may sometimes evolve to full-blown dementia. At this stage, delusions and hallucinations are frequently present, and their severity is significantly related to the dose of antiparkinsonian medication (i.e., the higher the dose, the greater the risk of psychotic behaviors). The dilemma then arises as to how to improve the patient's motor status while at the same time avoiding the risk of psychotic behaviors.

The past two decades witnessed an increasing number of investigations about the emotional, behavioral, and cognitive disorders in PD. To produce this book we had to go over hundreds of papers, sometimes with contradictory findings, with the need to address the complexities of the disease for the specialist, while at the same time allowing the text to remain accessible to the generalist. We hope that this goal was adequately met and that the book proves useful to a variety of mental-health-related professionals, such as neurologists, psychiatrists, geriatricians, general practitioners, psychologists, and social workers.

Finally, we would like to acknowledge our great mentors, Bob Robinson and Andy Lees, for all their encouragement and support during many years, as well as a number of excellent collaborators who helped with our research activities during the past 10 years. They are Gustavo Petracca, Eran Chemerinski, Janus Kremer, Lilia Canevaro, and Angel Cammarota. We also thank Jonathan Robinson for proof reading the book before its final edition. Last but not least, this book would never have reached its final stage without the great secretarial skills of our dear Laura Miguez.

Sergio E. Starkstein
Marcelo Merello

Introduction

Parkinson's disease (PD) is a frequent neurologic disorder among elderly individuals. Whereas the hallmark of the disease is the presence of abnormal movements, comorbid psychiatric and cognitive abnormalities are frequently found. The major aim for the present book was to include up-to-date information regarding the diagnosis, phenomenology, and treatment of the psychiatric and cognitive disorders of PD in one single volume.

Most patients with PD are usually cared for by internists and general practitioners, but the information about emotional and cognitive comorbid conditions is usually found in specialized neurologic and psychiatric journals. Our book is aimed at senior clinicians and trainees in internal medicine and general practice, at neurologists who may want a better understanding of their patients' "non-motor" problems, and at geriatric psychiatrists who may want to access the relevant information about emotion and cognition in PD, and update their knowledge about the motor complications and treatment of this disorder.

The second chapter provides a strong clinical background of the motor problems of PD before discussing the psychiatric and cognitive disorders related to the illness. We address the epidemiology and main clinical aspects of PD, and a clinical case is presented to illustrate the progression along the stages of the illness. There is also specific discussion of the different clinical complications that may emerge during the evolution of the disease and the subtypes of the illness. Treatment strategies for the motor disorder are specifically addressed, with discussion of emotional and cognitive benefits and complications of the different pharmacologic approaches such as the use of neuroprotective agents, levodopa (l-dopa) and dopaminergic agonists, anticholinergics, and other compounds. This chapter also includes a review of the most recent surgical treatments for PD, such as the stereotaxic lesion or stimulation of the posteroventral-pallidum, the thalamus, and the subthalamic nucleus, with special emphasis on the potential cognitive and emotional implications of these techniques.

In the third chapter we revise the most important differential diagnoses of PD to help the clinician understand diagnostic dilemmas of the disease. We provide clinical vignettes and discuss clinical aspects and laboratory and neuropathologic findings of multisystem atrophy, progressive supranuclear palsy, and corticobasal degeneration. Special attention is given to the spectrum of Lewy body disease, and clues for the differential diagnosis between PD and other neurodegenerative conditions, drug-induced parkinsonism, and parkinsonism related to depression, stroke, and "cortical" dementias are also provided.

In the fourth chapter we discuss the most frequent cognitive deficits in PD such as deficits in executive functions, visuospatial abilities, speech, language, attention, and memory. We examine their prevalence, potential mechanisms, and neuroimaging correlates. There is also an in-depth discussion of dementia in PD. After presenting a clinical vignette, we discuss methodologic issues related to the diagnosis of dementia in PD, and review the prevalence and phenomenology of dementia in this disorder. We specifically review cognitive, emotional, motor, and neuroimaging differences between so-called "subcortical" dementias (e.g., PD) and "cortical" dementias (e.g., Alzheimer's disease (AD)), and revise the clinical correlates and mechanism of dementia in PD. Specific reference is made to neuropathologic aspects of dementia in PD, such as coexisting AD pathology, cortical Lewy bodies, and depletion of neurotransmitter systems.

In the fifth chapter we examine the prevalence and phenomenology of depression in PD. We discuss the main strategies used to diagnose an affective disorder among patients with a neurologic disorder that may "mimic" a depressive condition, and we revise the main psychiatric instruments and diagnostic criteria used to carry out the patient's evaluation. We then discuss the impact of depression upon cognitive functioning, activities of daily living, quality of life, and evolution of the motor disorder. Finally, we examine biological markers and neuroimaging correlates of depression in PD and discuss potential underlying mechanisms for this condition.

In the sixth chapter we address behavioral disorders frequently reported in PD such as anxiety, panic attacks, phobias, and apathy. We discuss clues for the diagnosis of these problems and present illustrative cases. PD patients were reported as having "high moral standards," "moral exactitude," "great social conformism," and "inflexible social interactions." However, it was only recently that specific personality traits in PD have been investigated with standardized instruments. This chapter presents the main evidence for and against a specific personality "type" in PD.

In the seventh chapter we review the main cognitive and psychiatric side-effects of antiparkinsonian medication. We discuss the dilemma of improving the motor status of a patient while at the same time increasing the risk of behavioral problems, and examine alternatives for managing these difficult situations. The main psychiatric side-effects of antiparkinsonian medications are hallucinations, delusions, illusions, delirium, and sleep disorders. We examine their prevalence, main clinical correlates, and potential mechanisms. We then address the cognitive and emotional side-effects of specific antiparkinsonian drugs, such as l-dopa, dopaminergic agonists, amantadine, selegiline, and anticholinergic drugs.

In the eighth, and last, chapter we discuss the main somatic and psychological treatments of the psychiatric disorders of PD. The efficacy and side-effects of different types of antidepressants (e.g., tricyclics, mono-amine-oxidase inhibitors, selective serotonergic reuptake inhibitors) and antipsychotic agents (e.g., clozapine, risperidone, olanzapine, quetiapine) are specifically revised, and the usefulness of other treatment modalities, from relevant social and familial interventions to electroconvulsive therapy, is discussed.

Finally, the Appendix comprises seven scales that are frequently used to rate the physical and behavioral disorders of PD, as well as deficits in activities of daily living, and quality of life.

Epidemiologic, clinical, and therapeutic aspects of Parkinson's disease

Involuntary tremulous motion, with lessened muscular power, in parts not in action and even when supported, with a propensity to bend the trunk forwards, and to pass from a walking to a running pace: the senses and intellects being uninjured.

James Parkinson, 1817

Introduction

Since its initial description in 1817, PD remains an unsolved clinical problem, with a changing focus during the past four decades. Thus, the 1960s were the years of dopamine discovery; the 1970s witnessed a leap forward in the treatment of the disease by the introduction of replacement therapy with l-dopa; the 1980s witnessed motor complications emerging from chronic long-term l-dopa treatment; and the 1990s were primarily devoted to genetic and neuroimaging studies, the search for putative biological markers, and the rebirth of surgical treatment for the disease.

This chapter will examine relevant epidemiologic, clinical, and therapeutic aspects of PD and will provide the neurologic basis for the in-depth discussion of neuropsychiatric and cognitive aspects of the disease that follows.

Clinical vignette

A.B. is a 54-year-old accountant who noticed mild tremor in his right hand while reading the newspaper. A diagnosis of PD was made and the patient was started on l-dopa, which was followed by the disappearance of tremor. One year later, he noticed tremor during stressful situations, and his signature became smaller. He also noticed dragging of his right foot when walking. This overall picture illustrates the period of *stable response to l-dopa*.

Two years later, the patient developed clumsiness in both legs and abnormal gait. There was resting tremor in both hands, mostly in stressful situations. He had an abnormal flexed posture and lacked bilateral arm swing. The patient became less communicative in social situations and had a marked reduction in voice volume. The motor response to l-dopa was stable during the day, but he would wake up in the morning with bilateral tremor, difficulty in walking, and slowness while washing and shaving, followed by marked improvement 10–20 minutes after taking the first dose of l-dopa. This illustrates the period of *stable response with early morning akinesia*.

Two years later, despite an increase in l-dopa dosage and combination therapy with bromocriptine, the patient showed difficulties with most daily activities, as well as recurrence of tremor and other parkinsonian signs about 3–4 hours after taking l-dopa. His balance was normal but he was unsteady when turning around, and the frequency of l-dopa intake had to be increased. This illustrates the period of *fluctuating response with wearing-off phenomena*.

One year later, the patient became severely disabled in his daily activities. Nights were very uncomfortable due to increased rigidity. During the day he experienced a rapid decrease in medication efficacy: more than 30 minutes were necessary to "switch On" (i.e., to experience motor improvement), and "Off" periods (i.e., lack of motor improvement) lasted for more than 2 hours (e.g., he was totally disabled after lunch). Bromocriptine doses were progressively increased, but without a consistent motor improvement. He developed involuntary movements during the period of best medication effect, which were noticed by his wife but not by the patient himself. This illustrates the period of *fluctuating response with wearing-off phenomena, delayed On, poor response with empty stomach, and peak dose chorea*.

Two years later the patient was on a schedule of 800 mg l-dopa and 3 mg pergolide every 3 hours, but continued to experience wearing-off about 2–3 hours after medication intake. He was well aware of severe right-side involuntary movements, both at the beginning and at the end of each l-dopa dose. He also reported that the effect of medication would suddenly disappear during stressful situations, to return about 5–10 minutes later. Occasionally, the medication failed to switch him On, which mostly ocurred after meals. The patient developed severe postural instability during Off periods. He was unable to work, and needed assistance with most regular chores. This illustrates the period of *fluctuating response with wearing-off phenomena, the On–Off phenomenon, delayed On, poor response with empty stomach, failure of dose, and biphasic dyskinesias*.

Phenomenology of PD

Staging of illness

PD is a chronic and progressive disorder, which is usually divided into five different stages of severity (Table 2.1) (Hoehn & Yahr, 1967). As illustrated

Table 2.1. Modified Hoehn and Yahr staging of PD

Stage 0	No signs of disease
Stage 1	Unilateral disease
Stage 1.5	Unilateral disease plus axial involvement
Stage 2	Bilateral disease, without impaired balance
Stage 2.5	Bilateral disease, with recovery on pull test
Stage 3	Mild to moderate bilateral disease; some postural instability; physically independent
Stage 4	Severe disability; still able to walk or stand unassisted
Stage 5	Wheelchair-bound or bedridden unless aided

Adapted from Lang et al. (1995).

in the clinical vignette, stage I (i.e., stable response to l-dopa) is character-ized by symptoms exclusively or more prominently on one side of the body (Hughes et al., 1993). Parkinsonian signs such as tremor, rigidity, and bradykinesia may be confined to one side of the body for months or years, with a mean duration for this stage of about 3 years. Activities of daily living (ADLs) are usually not affected in this stage. Stage 2 (i.e., stable response with early morning akinesia) is characterized by spreading of parkinsonian signs to the opposite side of the body and to axial structures. During this stage the side initially affected still remains relatively more affected, but there is flexed posture with adduction of limbs, facial masking with monot-onous speech, mild disturbance of gait, generalized slowness, and a de-creased amplitude of associated movements. These signs are mostly mild, and balance is usually not affected. Stage 3 (i.e., fluctuating response with wearing-off phenomena) is characterized by impairment of balance and abnormal postural reflexes. Patients walk unsteadily and have difficulties when turning around. When pushed, patients may take several steps back-wards to maintain upright posture, and may fall. During this stage patients are functionally independent in household chores, but may show some limitations at work. Stage 4 (i.e., fluctuating response and On–Off phenom-ena) is characterized by increasing disabilities and partial dependence for most ADLs such as eating, dressing, and washing. All cardinal symptoms of the disease are markedly worse. During stage 5, the last of the illness, patients are completely dependent in their ADLs and restricted to a wheel-chair or bed bound. They require constant nursing care, and the main cause of death is aspirative pneumonia (Morgante et al., 2000).

Before the introduction of l-dopa, the mean survival period after the onset of parkinsonian signs was 10 years, and the rate of observed mortality was three times that of the general population (Hoehn & Yahr, 1967). Following l-dopa introduction, life expectancy increased by a mean of 6 years (Yahr, 1976).

Clinical features

The cardinal signs of PD are resting tremor, rigidity, bradykinesia, and loss of postural reflexes. We will now address each of these signs separately.

Resting tremor

A 3–5 Hz hand tremor ("pill rolling" tremor) is usually the initial symptom of the disease, and becomes most evident when hands are at rest. Parkinsonian tremor usually dampens during action or with support, but some PD patients may also show action tremor. Lower lip or chin tremor is not uncommon, but leg tremor is less frequent. Patients may show increased resting tremor when performing activities with the contralateral hand, during effortful thinking, and while walking.

Rigidity

Parkinsonian rigidity is characterized by a constant resistance to passive movement ("lead pipe" rigidity). Patients usually describe a stiff feeling, and rigidity may be elicited during physical examination. A ratchety catching known as "cogwheeling" may be felt when wrists are passively rotated, or while moving the arms at the elbow and the legs at the knee. Cogwheeling results from a combination of rigidity and tremor, and is not specific to parkinsonism (Kurlan et al., 2000).

Bradykinesia

This term is used to refer to slowness of movement or impaired initiation of movement, whereas hypokinesia or akinesia refer to poor movement or lack of movement. This symptom is usually the most disabling to patients.

Postural instability

PD patients have problems in standing up from a sitting position, maintaining postural stability, and adopting an erect posture. Patients may lose balance spontaneously or prove unable to maintain balance when pulled backwards. About one-third of PD patients have frequent falls.

PD patients may also show a diversity of additional motor symptoms, which are mostly variants of the cardinal signs described above. Hypomimia, or loss of facial expression, also termed "*masked face*," is most likely to be the result of combined bradykinesia and rigidity, and *dysarthria, hypophonia, and sialorrhea* may have a similar mechanism. Other manifestations of bradykinesia are *micrographia, decreased blink rate, loss of arm swing, and shuffling gait.* Respiratory problems are frequent and mostly result from respiratory muscle restriction due to rigidity. Other frequent findings are *blepharospasm* (i.e., involuntary bilateral eye closure produced by spasmodic contraction of the orbicularis oculi muscles), the "*striatal*" *hand* (i.e., a hand deformity often confused with rheumatoid arthritis), *foot deformity, and scoliosis* (Hartman & Abbs, 1988; Jankovic, 1987; Kurland et al., 1987; Logemann, 1988; Sudarsky & Ronthal, 1983; Weiner et al., 1984). A variety of oculomotor abnormalities have been described in PD patients, such as visual contrast deficits, upgaze limitation, abnormalities in smooth pursuit and vestibulo-ocular reflexes, decreased blink rate, positive glabellar reflex, eyelid aperture apraxia, and hypometric saccades (White et al., 1981).

The following non-motor clinical signs may also be frequently present in PD.

Autonomic dysfunction

This disorder may result from the disease itself or from antiparkinsonian drugs, and includes constipation, excessive saliva production, excessive perspiration, bowel dysfunction, impotence, loss of libido, and hyposmia.

Orthostasis

Orthostatic hypotension is a reduction in systolic blood pressure of at least 20 mmHg or a reduction in diastolic blood pressure of at least 10 mmHg, within 3 minutes of standing. Symptomatic or asymptomatic orthostatic hypotension may be present in up to 15% of normal elderly subjects, but the presence of severe orthostatic hypotension and other autonomic signs suggests alternative diagnoses to PD, such as multiple system atrophy (Hughes et al., 1993).

Dementia

Cognitive impairment commonly develops in a large proportion of parkinsonian patients. This subject is further discussed in chapter 4.

Depression

Depressive mood is present in about 40% of cross-sectional samples of PD patients, and most PD patients may show depression at some point in their longitudinal evolution. This issue is further discussed in chapter 5.

Psychotic features

Hallucinations, delusions, and illusions occur in about 40% of parkinsonian patients on dopamine replacement therapy, but are uncommon as a manifestation of the disease itself. This subject is further discussed in chapter 7.

Clusters of parkinsonian signs and subgroups of the disease

A question now arising is whether PD constitutes one single and clinically homogeneous disorder, or whether it should be considered as a generic term that covers a variety of somewhat related clinical subgroups. Based on the clinical heterogeneity of PD, several authors proposed subgroups with specific clinical characteristics (Zetusky et al., 1985). The identification of subgroups may be useful provided that this classification predicts genetic risk, associated clinical complications, rate of progression, or response to treatment. Zetusky et al. (1985) used the term "classical-PD" to refer to those patients with tremor as the predominant parkinsonian sign. This type of PD has a relatively early onset, relatively mild bradykinesia and postural instability, a relatively low prevalence of dementia, and a relatively higher likelihood of a positive family history of either PD or postural tremor. The second type of PD was termed "akinetic–rigid", and is characterized by a relatively high prevalence of dementia, depression, postural instability, and gait disorders.

Several authors (Barbeau & Roy, 1982; Quinn et al., 1987; Yokochi & Narabayashi, 1981) separated an "early" from a "late" onset form of PD. The current consensus is to use the term "early-onset" PD whenever parkinsonian signs develop before 40 years of age. This group is further subdivided into a "juvenile" type, whenever parkinsonian signs develop

Table 2.2. Most prevalent motor fluctuations in PD

Short-lasting motor fluctuations
Paradoxic kinesis
Freezing gait
On–Off

Medium-lasting motor fluctuations
Beginning of dose motor deterioration
End of dose motor deterioration
Wearing-off
On–Off
Yo-yoing
Diurnal fluctuation
Sleep benefit

Long-lasting motor fluctuations
Menstrual fluctuations

Adapted from Quinn (1999).

before 21 years of age, and an "adult" type, whenever parkinsonian signs develop between 21 and 39 years of age. Juvenile-type PD was reported to have a strong genetic component (Pineda-Trujillo et al., 2001), whereas early-onset, adult-type PD usually shows dystonia as the initial symptom, and dyskinesias and motor fluctuations relatively early after the onset of illness. Finally, the term "late-onset" PD is used whenever parkinsonian signs develop after 40 years of age, and is the most frequent type of PD.

Motor fluctuations

Motor fluctuations are considered to be an inevitable result of long-term l-dopa therapy, and may produce severe disability. Motor fluctuations may disrupt daily activities, and may occur together with fluctuations in mood and in sensory and autonomic functions (Table 2.2). About half of the patients with PD develop motor fluctuations and dyskinesias at some point during the illness (Sweet & McDowell, 1975). Several factors, such as l-dopa dose and age at onset of motor signs, may influence the rate of motor complications in PD. After a 6-year treatment period, patients on a low-dose l-dopa regimen (< 500 mg/day) were reported to show a prevalence of motor fluctuations of 52% and a prevalence of dyskinesias of 54%, whereas patients on high doses of l-dopa (> 1000 mg/day) were reported to show a higher prevalence of motor fluctuations and dyskinesias (80% and 88%, respectively) (Poewe et al., 1986). Kostic et al. (1991) reported that 96% of their series of patients with onset of PD before 40 years of age developed motor fluctuations, compared with 64% of PD patients with onset of parkinsonism after 40 years of age, supporting a significant association between early-onset PD and a greater risk of developing motor fluctuations.

Motor fluctuations related to l-dopa

L-dopa may produce three different motor responses: (1) A *short-term response*, which consists of a motor improvement that roughly parallels the increasing plasma l-dopa level and ends in a peak motor response; (2) a *long-term response*, which consists of a slowly increasing motor improvement that deteriorates over several days; and (3) an *inhibitory response* ("super Off"), which consists of a motor deterioration following or preceding the short-term response, and which may last from a few minutes to up to one hour (Nutt et al., 1988, 1997a, 1997b; Merello & Lees, 1992). All three motor responses are superimposed on a diurnal pattern of motor function, which is independent of l-dopa therapy and which is characterized by improved morning performance due to sleep benefit and declining evening function (Currie et al., 1997; Merello et al., 1997).

Types of motor fluctuations

Stable motor response

A stable response is defined as an l-dopa-related improvement of motor function in the absence of motor fluctuations in patients on less than five daily doses of l-dopa. This response is typically observed during the early course of the disease and may last for several years. A stable response occurs whenever a short-term response to a single l-dopa dose provides sustained motor benefit and overlaps with both the previous and following doses.

Wearing-off

Wearing-off is the return of parkinsonian signs at the end of the l-dopa dose cycle, and results from the progressive decline of the short-term response.

Early morning akinesia is the earliest sign of wearing-off and is produced by overnight l-dopa withdrawal. Beginning and end of dose "rebounds" are negative responses (i.e., more severe parkinsonian signs) that may occur at the beginning or end of each l-dopa cycle (Nutt et al., 1988; Merello & Lees, 1992).

On–off phenomenon

The so-called "On–Off" motor fluctuation is a rapid switching from On to Off states, which mostly occurs in advanced cases of PD (Nutt et al., 1984, 1992). "Yo-Yoing" consists of a chaotic fluctuation between On and Off states, which usually occurs in patients receiving complex l-dopa dosing schedules.

Dyskinesias

Dyskinesias are involuntary choreic, ballistic, or dystonic movements elicited by l-dopa or dopamine agonists. Dyskinesias occurring during the On state are termed "peak-of-dose." These abnormal movements are usually triggered by motor activity or stress, and may decrease with motor relaxation and inactivity. Some patients may experience dyskinesias both at the beginning and end of an l-dopa dose cycle, which is known as "biphasic dyskinesia."

Prevalence and etiology of PD

Parkinson's disease is a common disorder with a prevalence of 85–187 cases per 100 000 individuals (Brewis et al., 1966; Jenkins, 1966; Tanner et al., 1987) and an annual incidence of 12.4 cases per 100 000 women and 16.2 cases per 100 000 men (Tanner et al., 1987). Incidence rates for PD were found to increase with age in both sexes (Bower et al., 2000).

The etiology of PD remains unknown, but several mechanisms have been proposed. PD was considered to be a manifestation of accelerated aging (McGeer et al., 1977; Koller et al., 1986), but most available evidence suggests that PD is not simply an exacerbation of the normal aging process and is not explained by age-related brain changes (Gibb & Lees, 1987). Consistent evidence suggests that PD may result from free radical toxicity produced by oxidative reactions (Foley & Riederer, 2000). Free radicals generated by the oxidative metabolism of dopamine have an immediate reaction with membrane lipids, causing lipid peroxidation, membrane injury, and cell death. The compound, 1-methyl-4-phenyl-1,2,3,6-tetrahydropyridine (MPTP), is a self-injected drug used by addicts which may cause a clinical syndrome almost indistinguishable from PD, and is the best example of an environmental cause of parkinsonism (Langston & Ballard, 1984). The role of oxidation in the mechanism of PD was further strengthened by the finding of high levels of iron in the substantia nigra of PD patients (Becker & Berg, 2001). This mineral is known to facilitate oxidation and to decrease levels of glutathione, a chemical that protects against free radical formation. Several population studies demonstrated a higher prevalence of PD in industrialized countries compared with agricultural communities (Masalha et al., 1997). Other studies reported a significant association between PD and long-term consumption of well water, or between PD and working with industrial pesticides (Semchuk et al., 1992; Gorell et al., 1999; Racette et al., 2001).

Less than a century after James Parkinson's original description, Gowers (1896) suggested a familial aggregation for PD in some of his patients, but the role of genetics in PD remained a controversial issue for decades. During the last 10 years, several authors reported pedigrees of PD patients with a dominant pattern of inheritance (Kurland, 1958; Hoehn & Yahr, 1967; Duvoisin, 1984). A recent multivariate analysis demonstrated a family history of PD to be the main independent risk factor for the disease (Werneck & Alvarenga, 1999), and several uncontrolled studies reported frequencies of PD in first-degree relatives of probands with PD ranging between 2% and 47% (Barbeau & Roy, 1982). However, the genetic pattern of PD is not homogeneous, and may include age-related non-penetrance and complex segregation of traits from multiple loci (Polymeropoulos, 2000). A recent study reported a significantly increased risk of PD in carriers of the APOE-2 allele, and the presence of at least one E2 allele was found to multiply the risk for developing dementia in patients with PD (Harhangi et al., 2000).

Neuroimaging correlates of PD

Metabolic activity in the basal ganglia, and dopaminergic neurotransmission, have been extensively examined in PD using positron emission tomography (PET) and single photon emission computed tomography (SPECT). Metabolic and cerebral blood flow studies using [^{18}F] fluorodeoxyglucose or [Tc 99m] hexamethylpropylene-amine oxime, for PET and SPECT studies respectively, only showed discrete or no abnormalities in the basal ganglia, and non-specific cortical hypometabolism or hypoperfusion (Acton & Mozley, 2000). PET studies that assessed the integrity of dopamine neurons, using the uptake of [^{18}F] fluorodopa, demonstrated a significant low binding in the basal ganglia of PD patients (Garnett et al., 1983). This binding is related to the indemnity of striatal dopaminergic terminals, which are proportional to the number of dopamine neurons in the substantia nigra. Recent imaging studies measured the density of dopamine D2 receptors and reported a significant neuronal depletion in the basal ganglia of PD patients (putamen greater than caudate) (Tatsch et al., 1997). Studies with SPECT and [^{123}I] β-CIT demonstrated a 100% accuracy in distinguishing between PD patients and healthy controls using quantitative image analysis (Seibyl et al., 1995). Whereas PET and SPECT imaging studies may easily distinguish PD patients from healthy controls, there is an important loss of specificity whenever PD patients are compared with patients with other neurodegenerative disorders (see chapter 3 for further discussion).

PET and SPECT techniques were also used to measure the rate of progression of PD, and most studies showed the rate of depletion of dopaminergic neurons to be significantly greater in PD compared with the normal aging process (Morrish et al., 1998). Based on these studies, the onset of parkinsonian signs was estimated to occur after a decline of dopaminergic neurons of about 75% for the putamen, and 91% for the caudate (Morrish et al., 1998).

Neuropathologic correlates of PD

A pathologic diagnosis of idiopathic PD requires the presence of depigmentation and neuronal loss in the compact zone of the substantia nigra, together with intraneuronal filamentous inclusions known as Lewy bodies. Recent work has shown that these Lewy bodies are made of the protein alpha-synuclein (Spillantini & Goedert, 2000). About 60–75% of cases with a clinical diagnosis of PD may meet the neuropathologic criteria for PD, whereas the remaining cases will show other pathologies such as multiple system atrophy, progressive supranuclear palsy, Alzheimer's disease, or cerebrovascular lesions. The United Kingdom Parkinson's Disease Society Brain Bank clinical diagnostic criteria (Hughes et al., 1993) were found to have a specificity of 82% for neuropathologically confirmed PD (Table 2.3).

Lewy bodies are also frequent in the locus coeruleus, the dorsal motor vagus nucleus, the substantia innominata, the hypothalamus, and the amygdala, and cortical Lewy bodies may be found in about 10% of PD patients (Lewy, 1912, 1923; Forno, 1987). However, Lewy bodies are not specific for PD and may also be found in patients with other neurologic disorders, such as Alzheimer's disease, post-encephalitic parkinsonism, infantile neuroaxonal dystrophy, ataxia-telangiectasia, and subacute leukoencephalopathy (Agamanolis & Greenstein, 1979; Forno, 1987).

Mechanisms of PD

Before discussing the potential mechanisms of PD, we will briefly review the anatomy and physiology of the basal ganglia, as well as the pharmacology of dopamine receptors.

The basal ganglia system

The basal ganglia are a group of hierarchically interconnected subcortical nuclei which play a major role in the modulation of motor and non-motor behaviors. The basal ganglia include the striatal complex, the globus pallidus, the substantia nigra, and the subthalamic nucleus. In primates and other mammals, the dorsal striatal complex is divided by the internal capsule into the caudate and the putamen. The ventral extensions of the medial and lateral striatal complex fuse into the nucleus accumbens and the olfactory tubercle. In primates, the globus pallidus is divided into an internal (GPi) and an external (GPe) segment, and the substantia nigra is subdivided into the densely packed pars compacta (SNc) and the less dense pars reticulata (SNr) (Parent & Hazrati, 1995).

The basal ganglia participate in corticobasal ganglionic-thalamocortical loops, which collect information from a broad array of forebrain structures, "funnel" it through the basal ganglia, and route it back to the cortex via specific thalamic relays. The striatal complex receives massive input from

Table 2.3. UK Parkinson's Disease Society Brain Bank clinical diagnostic criteria for PD

Step 1: Diagnosis of parkinsonism

1. Bradykinesia
2. At least one of the following: (a) Rigidity, (b) rest tremor or postural instability (not related to visual, vestibular, cerebellar, or proprioceptive dysfunction)

Step 2: Exclusion criteria for PD

1. History of repeated strokes with stepwise progression of parkinsonian signs
2. History of repeated head injury
3. History of encephalitis
4. Oculogyric crises
5. Neuroleptic treatment at symptom onset
6. More than one affected relative
7. Sustained remission
8. Strictly unilateral signs after 3 years since onset
9. Supranuclear gaze palsy
10. Cerebellar signs
11. Early severe autonomic dysfunction
12. Early severe initial dementia with apraxia
13. Extensor plantar response
14. Cerebral tumor or hydrocephalus on CT scan
15. Negative response to l-dopa (more than 1 g during more than 1 month)
16. MPTP exposure

Step 3: Supportive prospective positive criteria for PD

(at least three are necessary for definite diagnosis)

1. Unilateral onset
2. Rest tremor
3. Progressive disorder
4. Persistent asymmetry of parkinsonism
5. Marked response to l-dopa/apomorphine
6. Severe l-dopa-induced dyskinesias
7. L-dopa responsiveness for more than 5 years
8. Duration of illness of 10 years or more

Adapted from Hughes et al. (1992).

the neocortical mantle, the hippocampal formation, the amygdala, the primary olfactory cortex, and the midline thalamic nuclei. These inputs are mostly excitatory and use the neurotransmitter glutamate. Approximately 90–95% of striatal neurons have inhibitory GABA-ergic axons which terminate in both internal and external segments of the globus pallidus and in both components of the substantia nigra. The GPi and the SNr are the primary output relay stations of the basal ganglia and may be considered as a single functional unit. Both the GPi and SNr consist of GABA-ergic inhibitory neurons which mostly project to the mediodorsal thalamic nuclei, but which also send projections to the superior colliculus, the lateral habenula, and the pedunculopontine nucleus. In turn, the thalamic nuclei project to specific cortical regions such as the primary motor, premotor, and prefrontal cortices. This cortico-subcortical system includes a number of subsidiary loops mostly involving the SNc and the subthalamic nucleus (STN). The SNc receives a dense GABA-ergic innervation from the striatum and sends dopaminergic efferents back to the striatum. The STN receives a major GABA-ergic inhibitory input from the GPe, and projects excitatory glutamatergic efferents to both segments of the globus pallidus, to both components of the substantia nigra, and to the striatum itself (Figure 2.1).

Pharmacology of dopamine receptors

Up to this writing, a total of five subtypes of dopamine receptors have been cloned, which were grouped into D_1-like (including D_1 and D_5 receptors) and D_2-like (including D_2, D_3, and D_4 receptors) families. Dopamine receptors are encoded into different genes: The D_1 receptor gene is on chromosome 5, the D_2 and D_4 receptor genes are on chromosome 11, the D_3 receptor gene is on chromosome 3, and the D_5 receptor gene is on chromosome 4 (Grandy et al., 1989; Le Coniat et al., 1991; Sunahara et al., 1991; Tiberti et al., 1991; van Tol et al., 1991). D_1 and D_2 receptors are mostly localized in the striatum and in the substantia nigra. They are primarily post-synaptic receptors, although D_2 receptors are also pre-synaptic and regulate dopamine synthesis and release, and the rate of neuronal firing (Sokoloff et al., 1990). D_3 receptors are largely expressed in the ventral striatum and nucleus accumbens, D_4 receptors are expressed in the frontal

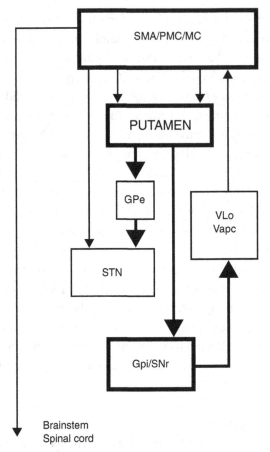

Figure 2.1. Normal brain cortico-subcortical connections (SMA, supplementary motor area; PMC, premotor cortex; MC, motor cortex; GPe, external globus pallidus; STN, subthalamic nucleus; GPi, internal globus pallidus; SNr, substantia nigra pars reticulata; VLo, ventral lateral thalamus, pars oralis; Vapc, ventral anterior thalamus, pars centralis).

cortex, and D_5 receptors are mostly localized in the mammillary and pretectal nuclei (Poewe & Granata, 1997).

Neurochemical mechanism

PD is characterized by dopaminergic denervation at both post-synaptic and pre-synaptic levels. At advanced stages of denervation (i.e., exceeding 90% of dopaminergic cell loss) there is up-regulation of post-synaptic D_1 and D_2

receptors (Gnanalingham et al., 1993), which is potentially reversible upon administration of l-dopa or other dopaminergic drugs. On the other hand, D_1 striatal receptors remain relatively unaffected during the illness (Rinne et al., 1990).

Parkinsonian motor signs are secondary to impaired dopamine function within the striatum, which may result from either loss of dopaminergic afferents to the striatum (such as in idiopathic or MPTP-induced PD), dopamine receptor blockade (as produced by some anti-psychotics and anti-emetics), or dopamine depletion (as produced by compounds such as reserpine, tetrabenazine, or alpha-methyldopa). Disruption of striatal dopamine function produces increased activity in striatal neuron sub-populations, followed by a cascade of events in other basal ganglia nuclei. Dopamine inhibits striato-GPe neurons and stimulates striato-GPi/SNr projection neurons, which may be related to the differential distribution of D_1 and D_2 receptors in these striatal projection neurons. Dopamine depletion produces abnormal function of corticostriatal inputs to striatal (mainly striato-GPe) projection neurons, which become more active and produce a concomitant decrease of activity in the striato-GPi/SNr circuit. This, in turn, produces both an increased inhibition of GPe neurons and a disinhibition of GPi and SNr neurons. The increased inhibition of GPe neurons results in both disinhibition of the STN and excessive excitatory drive to the GPi/SNr. Finally, the excessive GPi/SNr output to the thalamus produces an increased inhibition of thalamocortical projection neurons, and cortical hypoactivation (Figure 2.2).

Several imaging studies demonstrated significant hypoactivity in the mesial premotor and prefrontal areas in PD patients compared with healthy controls, which may be related to dopamine deficits in those brain areas and which may underlie akinesia in PD (Sabatini et al., 2000). Rascol et al. (1992) reported impaired motor activation in the mesial premotor cortex in PD, which may normalize after l-dopa medication. Haslinger et al. (2001) demonstrated increased bilateral activation within the lateral premotor cortex in PD compared with healthy controls, and speculated that PD may use the lateral premotor cortex to compensate for the hypofunction in striatofrontal dopaminergic projections.

The beneficial effect of dopaminergic drugs on PD motor symptoms is mostly related to D_2-like receptor stimulation, but D_1 receptor co-

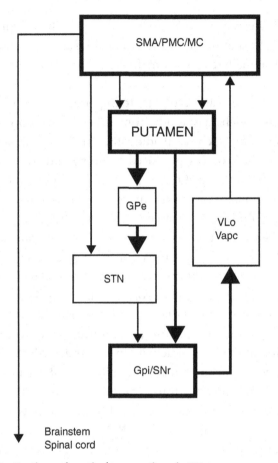

Figure 2.2. Cortico-subcortical connections in PD.

stimulation was also found to reverse parkinsonian motor deficits (Bédard et al., 1997).

Treatment of PD

The major therapeutic goal in PD is to tailor treatment to each patient in order to maintain maximal function. Thus, the strategy to treat a young PD patient should take into account several factors liable to affect long-term prognosis, and may differ substantially from the therapeutic approach to an

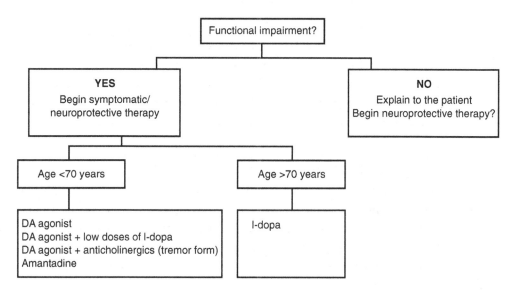

Figure 2.3. The pharmacologic treatment of PD.

elderly PD patient, for whom there is less concern over "neuroprotection" and more towards symptomatic relief. We will now review the most accepted treatment modalities for the different stages of PD and types of dysfunction (Figure 2.3).

Neuroprotective agents

Selegiline is a monoamine oxidase B (MAO-B) inhibitor that is reported to delay the progression of the disease (Parkinson Study Group, 1989). However, no long-term benefits of this drug could be demonstrated (Parkinson Study Group, 1990), and there is no convincing evidence that vitamin E or other types of antioxidants may slow down the progression of PD. The use of selegiline combined with l-dopa was reported to be associated with greater mortality than the use of l-dopa alone (Ben-Shlomo et al., 1998, but see Donnan et al., 2000, for a different outcome), and to produce a significantly higher risk of cardiovascular adverse reactions (Montastruc et al., 2000).

Anticholinergics

Drugs that block central muscarinic acetylcholine receptors such as trihexyphenidyl, procyclidine, orphenadrine, and benztropine were shown to improve resting tremor in PD and are mostly used in young patients (Hristova & Koller, 2000). Treatment starts with low doses, which are gradually increased until symptomatic relief is obtained. Unfortunately, treatment is often accompanied by frequent and sometimes severe side-effects such as dry mouth, blurred vision, confusion, and memory loss, and nowadays these compounds are rarely used.

N-methyl-D-aspartate (NMDA) blockers

Amantadine is an adamantane derivative which exerts its action by NMDA central receptor blocking and which also has anticholinergic effects. Amantadine may produce short-term symptomatic benefit in the early stages of illness, and may be useful to treat drug-induced dyskinesias in patients on long-term treatment with l-dopa (Goetz, 1998; Luginger et al., 2000). Amantadine should be started at 100 mg/day and slowly increased until a dose of 300 mg/day. Most frequent side-effects are nausea and vomiting, but rare cases with hallucinations, lower limb oedema, and livedo reticularis were also reported.

Memantine is another NMDA blocker that was reported to have some antiparkinsonian effect in advanced cases of PD (Merello et al., 1999b). Initial doses are 10 mg/day which may be increased to up to 30 mg/day, and most frequent side-effects are insomnia and nervousness.

L-dopa

L-dopa is a neutral amino acid which is converted to dopamine and other metabolites. A combination of l-dopa with a dopa-decarboxylase inhibitor such as carbidopa or benserazide remains the most effective symptomatic treatment for PD. L-dopa is converted to dopamine by central dopa-decarboxylase, stored in dopamine neurons, and released to the synaptic space to act on dopamine receptors. Carbidopa and benserazide are peripheral inhibitors of dopa-decarboxylase, which reduce the severity of side-effects of l-dopa such as hypotension, tachycardia, nausea, and vomiting, and allow more l-dopa to cross the blood–brain barrier. There are three formulations of l-dopa: The standard formulation, which comes in different doses, a slow-release formulation, and a "fast-relief" dispersable preparation.

Dopamine agonists

Dopamine agonists such as bromocriptine, lisuride, and pergolide have a direct action on post-synaptic dopamine receptors and were initially used as adjuvants to l-dopa (Bedard et al., 1997). Later, several studies suggested a role for these compounds in the treatment of "de novo" PD patients (i.e., patients who had never received pharmacotherapy for PD). We will now address each of these compounds in more detail.

Bromocriptine mesylate

This is a D_2 agonist with partial D_1 antagonist activity in nanomolar concentrations, or partial D_1 agonist activity in micromolar concentrations (Schachter et al., 1980), with proven efficacy in treating PD (Lees & Stern, 1981). Bromocriptine monotherapy was reported to produce significantly fewer dyskinesias and motor fluctuations later in the disease compared with l-dopa (Lees & Stern, 1981; Parkinson's Disease Research Group in the United Kingdom, 1993; Monstastruc et al., 1994). On the other hand, bromocriptine provides less symptomatic improvement and has worse tolerability as compared to conventional l-dopa therapy (Parkinson's Disease Research Group in the United Kingdom, 1993). The addition of l-dopa to bromocriptine monotherapy may produce adequate symptomatic improvement and less l-dopa-induced dyskinesias than treatment with l-dopa alone (Montastruc et al., 1994). Bromocriptine was reported to reduce the "wearing-off" and "On–Off" fluctuations when associated with l-dopa and may also reduce l-dopa requirements by about 10–40% (Lieberman et al., 1983). When given together with l-dopa, bromocriptine doses usually range from 15 mg to 25 mg (Bromocriptine Research Group, 1989).

Lisuride hydrogen maleate

This is a semisynthetic ergot alkaloid with D_2 agonist and partial D_1 antagonist activity. Lisuride was reported to improve parkinsonian signs and reduce motor fluctuations when added to l-dopa (Rinne, 1989). Like bromocriptine, add-on therapy with lisuride allows an important l-dopa dose reduction, with a concomitant reduction in the frequency of peak-dose dyskinesias. In contrast to other available dopamine agonists, lisuride is readily soluble in water, allowing parenteral administration. However, continuous subcutaneous lisuride infusion with portable mini-pumps in patients with severe motor fluctuations was reported to produce a high prevalence of delirium and is no longer used (Vaamonde et al., 1991).

Pergolide mesylate

This is a semisynthetic ergot derivative, which is about 10 times more potent than bromocriptine and with a longer half-life (Rubin et al., 1981). Pergolide stimulates both D_1 and D_2 receptors, and has high affinity for D_3 receptors (Sokoloff et al., 1990). Pergolide was reported to reduce motor fluctuations by over 30%, allowing a reduction of concomitant l-dopa dose of about 25% (Langtry & Clissold, 1990; Reinmuth et al., 1994). A comparison between pergolide and bromocriptine as add-on drugs in l-dopa-treated patients with fluctuating response and dyskinesias demonstrated a somewhat better efficacy and tolerability for pergolide (Lieberman et al., 1983; Goetz et al., 1985).

Apomorphine

This is a potent D_1 and D_2 agonist with robust antiparkinsonian effects. This drug has poor bioavailability when given orally due to an extensive first-pass effect, but is readily absorbed after sublingual, intranasal or rectal administration. Subcutaneous bolus injections or continuous subcutaneous infusions of apomorphine were reported to be highly effective in reducing motor fluctuations and Off periods (Stibe et al., 1988; Frankel et al., 1990). PD patients with unpredictable and frequent On–Off fluctuations or l-dopa-related dyskinesias were reported to benefit from continuous subcutaneous apomorphine infusions delivered through portable minipumps (Poewe, 1993). Frequent side-effects of apomorphine are nausea, vomiting, and hypotension. Red, itchy nodules at injection sites are frequently present, but are usually well tolerated and transient. Less frequent side-effects are sedation, visual hallucinations, and autoimmune hemolytic anemia. Monthly blood counts are mandatory.

Cabergoline

This is an ergot derivative with D_2 agonist activity, and a half-life exceeding 24 hours. Several studies demonstrated a longer action for this compound compared with bromocriptine, and adequate efficacy of single daily dose schedules (Inzelberg et al., 1996; Rinne et al., 1997).

Ropinirole

This compound has a high affinity for both D_2 and D_3 receptors, relatively less activity for D_4 receptors, and almost no activity for α-adrenergic or 5-HT receptors. A 5-year follow-up study demonstrated a relatively low prevalence of motor fluctuations associated with the use of ropinirole (Rascol et al., 2000).

Pramipexole

This compound is three times more potent than bromocriptine on dopaminergic receptors on a milligram-to-milligram basis. It lacks D_1 activity, and has some stimulatory effect at α_2-adrenoreceptors (Lieberman et al., 1997). Pramipexole was reported to allow a reduction of l-dopa dose and to improve Off period (Guttman, 1997), and somnolence is its most frequent side-effect (Hauser et al., 2000).

Catechol-O-methyl-transferase (COMT) inhibitors

COMT is the main catabolic pathway of l-dopa after dopa-decarboxylase inhibition. Tolcapone and entacapone are drugs that inhibit COMT, and recent studies demonstrated that these compounds prolong the duration of single doses of l-dopa and increase On time (Merello et al., 1994). Side-effects are mainly due to dopaminergic overstimulation and include dyskinesias, hallucinations, and nausea. Unfortunately, fulminant hepatitis was reported in three patients and tolcapone was withdrawn in several countries, while in others a weekly liver function test is mandatory.

Treatment of dyskinesias and motor fluctuations

The initial step in treating the motor complications of l-dopa therapy is to adjust doses and drug schedules to reduce the duration of the Off period. It is important to assess the pattern and duration of motor fluctuations, which may require the admission of the patient to the clinic, or the preparation of home charts to register the frequency and duration of On and Off periods. Motor fluctuations are often accompanied by autonomic and mood changes, which require their own specific treatment.

Frequent small doses of l-dopa may produce unpredictable responses and may increase motor fluctuations (Levy, 1966). Controlled-release l-dopa preparations have a relatively more erratic absorption than regular l-dopa, and in cases of unpredictable motor response, patients should be switched to regular l-dopa given 3–4 hours apart, but keeping the same total daily l-dopa dose. The addition of other antiparkinsonian agents at the time of l-dopa intake may help to produce a more predictable response.

The first step in reducing dyskinesias is to decrease adjuvant antiparkinsonian medication. Selegiline should be first tapered off and withdrawn, followed by switching of controlled-release l-dopa preparations to fast-release formulations, which may improve dyskinesias and enhance predictable motor responses. Although dopamine agonists rarely produce dyskinesias when given alone, these compounds may increase dyskinesias when added to l-dopa and may have to be discontinued in cases of severe dyskinesias and motor fluctuations. The next step is to lower l-dopa dose, although frequent small doses rarely prevent dyskinesias and may even increase the frequency of motor fluctuations. Amantadine and buspirone were both reported to reduce dyskinesias and increase the On period in some patients (Bonifati et al., 1994; Verhagen Metman et al., 1998). Finally, severely disabling dyskinesias may improve after pallidotomy contralateral to the most affected side.

In conclusion, l-dopa-related motor fluctuations and dyskinesias may complicate the management of PD and should be readily treated. These complications are strongly related to l-dopa intake, and l-dopa administration should be delayed until it becomes necessary to preserve overall function. L-dopa dosage may be reduced by adding other antiparkinsonian drugs. Starting treatment with dopamine agonists may postpone l-dopa requirements by 1–3 years, and may produce a lower rate of motor fluctuations and dyskinesias, although these abnormalities may appear as soon as l-dopa is started.

Surgical treatment

Whereas 30 years ago surgical treatment for PD was widely used, the introduction of l-dopa produced a rapid decline of this therapy. During the past decade there was a better understanding of the pathophysiological mechanisms of the disease, together with technological advances in neuro-imaging and electrophysiology and a renewed interest in surgical treatments for PD such as the implantation of dopamine-secreting cells. At present, the thalamus, the GPi, and the STN are the main targets of thermolesion or the implantation of electrodes for electrical stimulation. We will review the efficacy and main complications of each of these techniques.

Globus Pallidus

Motor effects of pallidotomy may depend upon the location of the lesion within the GPi, since lesions placed in the anterior section of the GPi were reported to produce greatest improvement of rigidity and l-dopa-induced dyskinesias, whereas more posterior lesions were reported to produce greatest decrease in tremor (Gross et al., 1999). Dogali et al. (1995) performed posteroventral pallidotomy (PVP) using a microrecording-guided technique in a series of 11 PD patients. One year after surgery there was a mean 65% decrement on the total Unified Parkinson's Disease Rating Scale (UPDRS) scores, a 38% decrease in contralateral severity and a 24% decrease in ipsilateral severity of rigidity, bradykinesia, and resting tremor, and a 45% increment in walking speed. Lozano et al. (1995) carried out posteroventral pallidotomy using the microrecording technique in 14 PD patients. At 6-month follow-up evaluation, there was a mean decrease of 30% on the UPDRS Off score, a 15% improvement on gait impairment, a 23% improvement on postural instability, and a 92% decrease in dyskinesia scores on the side contralateral to the pallidotomy. Surgical complications occurred in three patients, all of whom developed a mild slight facial paresis which lasted for about 3 weeks.

Lai et al. (2000) carried out PVP in a series of 89 patients with PD. Three months after surgery, 82% of the patients had a marked improvement in their parkinsonian signs, with a mean motor improvement in the Off state of 36% and a mean improvement in ADLs of 34%. These improvements were maintained 12 and 24 months after surgery. A recent study by Fine et al. (2000) reported improvements in the contralateral side of surgery to be sustained for up to $5\frac{1}{2}$ years after PVP. Merello et al. (1999a) compared the progression of parkinsonian symptoms in patients undergoing pallidotomy with non-operated PD patients with comparable disease severity. One year after surgery, the pallidotomy group showed reductions (i.e., improvements) in UPDRS scores of rigidity, tremor, and bradykinesia, whereas the non-operated PD group showed higher scores (i.e., worsening) in all three motor domains. There was also a significantly greater reduction in the frequency of dyskinesias in the operated group compared with the non-operated group of patients.

Pallidotomy was reported to produce visual field defects in about 4% of patients, whereas an additional 1.4% had permanent hemiparesis (Bronstein et al., 1999). Cognitive effects of unilateral PVP are usually mild and may depend on lesion location: more anterior pallidal lesions were reported to produce mild deficits in verbal fluency and calculation, medial lesions may not produce cognitive changes, and posterior lesions may even produce some cognitive improvement (Lombardi et al., 2000). Rettig et al. (2000) reported that patients with unilateral PVP showed significant improvements in confrontational naming and visuospatial organization up to 1 year after surgery, as well as a transient decline in verbal learning 3 months post surgery. Kuzis et al. (2001) assessed a series of 10 PD patients before, and 12 months after, unilateral PVP with a comprehensive neuropsychological battery. When this group was compared with 20 age- and disease-severity matched, non-operated PD patients with the same follow-up, no significant between-group differences were found on any cognitive measure. On the other hand, Stebbins et al. (2000) reported significant declines in tests of psychomotor processing speed, working memory, and reasoning (but not on measures of semantic memory) at 1-year follow-up in 11 PD patients who had PVP compared with a non-operated PD control group.

Bilateral PVP is rarely carried out as this procedure may produce significant side-effects such as speech, swallowing, and salivation difficulties, and severe behavioral changes (Ghika et al., 1998; Merello et al., 1999a). Indications and contraindications for PVP are provided in Table 2.4.

Deep-brain stimulation is a reversible, non-lesioning surgical treatment for PD, and consists of the implantation of a quadripolar electrode within the GPi, which is connected to a pulse generator implanted subcutaneously in the chest. Stimulation may inhibit the STN by excitation of inhibitory GABA-ergic neurons, and may also synchronize the STN discharge at a higher rate. Pahwa et al. (1997) placed stimulators in the GPi in six PD patients, and reported a significant improvement in cardinal symptoms of PD as well as a significant reduction in drug-induced dyskinesias after 3 months of stimulation. Merello et al. (1999c) carried out a randomized

Table 2.4. Indications and contraindications for posteroventral pallidotomy

Indications

Advanced disease with rigidity and bradykinesia, and a poor response to antiparkinsonian medications

Disabling dyskinesias

Severe motor fluctuations

Painful cramps and severe dystonias

Serious side-effects of antiparkinsonian medications

Contraindications

History of poor or no response to l-dopa treatment

History of strokes or other cerebral lesions

Severe cerebral atrophy

Coexistence of other diseases that impede adequate rehabilitation

Moderate to severe dementia

Adapted from Lai et al. (2000).

prospective study of unilateral posteroventral pallidotomy compared with unilateral posteroventral stimulation in 13 PD patients. Three months after surgery, there was a significant motor improvement in both groups, which was of a similar magnitude. Moreover, both treatments produced a similar rate of side-effects, which were mostly transient. Patients with bilateral parkinsonian signs may benefit from bilateral GPi inhibition, either by placing two stimulators in this structure, or by a combination of lesion on one GPi and a stimulator on the other (Galvez-Jimenez et al., 1998).

Side-effects of GPi stimulation were reported to be mild (Jahanshahi et al., 2000). However, Miyawaki et al. (2000) reported a patient who suffered transient episodes of mania and hypomania occurring after left, right or bilateral GPi stimulation. Confusion and focal cognitive dysfunction were reported during stimulation, and were reversed by adjustment of the stimulation parameters (Ghika et al., 1998; Dujardin et al., 2000). Other nonfrequent complications of this procedure include deep-brain hematomas and postoperative seizures. Stimulation may produce slight and transient paresthesias, dystonia contralateral to the electrode placement, postural imbalance, and dysarthria.

Thalamus

> Stereotaxic thalamic lesions were introduced as a treatment for PD about 50 years ago. These early studies reported improvement in tremor and rigidity of limbs contralateral to the thalamic lesion in over 90% of patients (Hassler et al., 1965). More recently, Kelly and Gillingham (1980) carried out unilateral thalamotomy in 57 PD patients: They reported no tremor in 90% and 57% of the patients 2 and 10 years after surgery, respectively. Nagasaki et al. (1986) found minimal recurrence of tremor after a 7-year follow-up in 27 PD patients who had unilateral thalamotomy, and a similar efficacy was reported by other authors. On the other hand, bradykinesia and tremor ipsilateral to the thalamotomy were reported not to improve (Nagasaki et al., 1986). The most frequent complications of thalamotomy are dysarthria and postural instability, but cognitive deficits are mild or absent (Hugdahl & Wester, 2000). Bilateral thalamotomy is no longer used due to the high frequency of severe side-effects.
>
> Benabid et al. (1991) demonstrated that stimulation of the ventral intermediate nucleus of the thalamus may produce significant improvements in tremor, but not in rigidity or bradykinesia. Ondo et al. (2001) demonstrated that bilateral thalamic stimulation is more effective than unilateral stimulation in improving bilateral appendicular and midline tremor in PD. The most frequent adverse effects of this technique are dysarthria, gait, and postural problems, and paresthesias, which are more frequent after bilateral compared with unilateral thalamic implantation (Ondo et al., 2001).

Subthalamic nucleus

> Small lesions in the caudomedial aspect of the STN may improve akinesia, tremor, and rigidity by reducing the outflow of excitatory activity from the STN to the GPi. Fager (1963) carried out unilateral STN lesions in five PD patients with severe gait freezing and axial akinesia. One of the patients suffered a large STN infarction and hemichorea 7 days after surgery. The other four patients had a significant improvement in tremor, rigidity, and bradykinesia, and were able to reduce their l-dopa dosage. McCarter et al. (2000) reported no global neuropsychological deficits relative to presurgical baseline in 12 PD patients who underwent subthalamic nucleotomy, although mild cognitive deficits were seen in some patients.
>
> Limousin et al. (1995) carried out bilateral STN stimulation in a 55-year-

old man with akinetic-rigid PD and severe motor fluctuations. Unilateral stimulation produced improvements in contralateral rigidity, akinesia, and Off-period dystonia, but there was no improvement on the side ipsilateral to surgery. Limousin et al. (1998) studied 24 PD patients with bilateral STN electrode implantations and long-term (1-year) stimulation. They found a 60% improvement in ADL scores, and significant improvements in limb akinesia, rigidity, tremor, and gait, which allowed a marked reduction in the dosage of dopaminergic agonists. Pillon et al. (2000) reported significant cognitive improvement in psychomotor speed and working memory when the STN stimulator was turned on, but no overall differences between STN and GPi stimulation were found in cognitive evaluation. Similar results were reported by Jahanshahi et al. (2000). STN stimulation was also reported to improve sleep problems in PD by reducing night-time akinesia and axial and early morning dystonia (Arnulf et al., 2000).

In conclusion, surgical lesions or electrical stimulation of the GPi were both reported to ameliorate the cardinal signs of PD and l-dopa-induced dyskinesias, mostly on the side contralateral to the surgical procedure (Table 2.5). These techniques are accepted treatments for patients with advanced disease for whom medication is not effective or is associated with disabling side-effects. Deep-brain stimulation consists of implanting electrodes in subcortical structures (e.g., GPi, STN) for chronic, high-frequency electrical stimulation. This effect is adaptable by changing clinical parameters, and proved to have a similar efficacy and fewer side-effects than PVP. Figure 2.4 provides an orienting algorithm for surgical therapies in PD.

General conclusions

PD is a chronic progressive disorder that evolves along five stages, from mild unilateral parkinsonian signs and a stable response to l-dopa in the initial stage, to complete dependency due to motor fluctuations, dyskinesias, and failure to respond to dopaminergic agents in late stages. The cardinal symptoms of PD are rigidity, bradykinesia, and resting tremor, but other frequent features of the disease are postural instability, autonomic dysfunction, dementia, and depression. About half of PD patients are completely disabled or dead after 10 years of illness. The neuropathology of

Table 2.5. Most relevant motor and pharmacologic effects of different surgical techniques for PD

	STN	GPi	VIM
Tremor	+++	++	+++
Bradykinesia	+++	+(+)	–
Rigidity	+++	+++	(+)
Dyskinesia	–/++	+++	(+)
Axial symptoms	+++	+	–
L-dopa dose reduction	+++	–	–
Off dystonia	+++	++	–

STN: subthalamic nucleus

GPi: internal globus pallidus

VIM: ventralic intermedius thalamic nucleus

Effect

+++ great improvement

++ moderate improvement

+ mild improvement

(+) questionable improvement

– no improvement

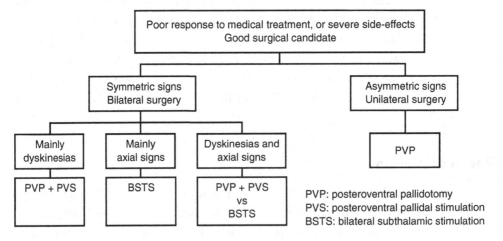

Figure 2.4. The surgical treatment of PD.

PD is characterized by neuronal loss and Lewy bodies in the compact zone of the substantia nigra, and pre- and post-synaptic dopaminergic denervation. L-dopa still remains the best treatment for PD and is usually started as an adjunct or as initial monotherapy in sustained-release preparations. Anticholinergic drugs may be used in young patients with tremor-dominant PD. It is not yet clear whether neuroprotective agents are useful in slowing down the progression of the illness. Dopamine agonists have an important role in the treatment of PD patients in the initial stages of the illness, and as adjuvants to l-dopa therapy. NMDA and COMT inhibitors demonstrated some efficacy, but experience is still limited. Surgical techniques, such as unilateral stereotaxic thermolesion of the globus pallidus, thalamus, or STN, or the implantation of stimulation electrodes in these structures, were found to produce significant clinical improvement, with little or no cognitive or motor sequelae.

Parkinsonism and Parkinson's disease

The diagnosis of PD requires a thorough investigation of the main neuro-logic signs of the disease, as well as the search for signs that are atypical of PD, which may suggest diferential diagnoses (Quinn, 1995). Several diag-nostic criteria for PD have been proposed (see Table 2.3), but even in the most experienced Movement Disorders Clinics, about 10–35% of patients initially diagnosed with PD will eventually be diagnosed with another disease (Rajput et al., 1991; Hughes et al., 1992a, 1992b) (Table 3.1).

Atypical parkinsonian disorders are characterized by parkinsonian signs (e.g., resting tremor, rigidity, and bradykinesia) and additional clinical manifestations that are atypical of PD, such as pyramidal, cerebellar, or autonomic signs (Table 3.2). The two most prevalent atypical parkinsonian disorders are progressive supranuclear palsy (Steele et al., 1964) and multiple system atrophy, and parkinsonism may be found in dementia with Lewy bodies (McKeith et al., 1996), secondary parkinsonism (Winikates & Jankovic, 1999), and less frequently, corticobasal degeneration (Rebeiz et al., 1968), Alzheimer's disease (Merello et al., 1994), Pick's disease (Brion et al., 1991), Parkinson-dementia-complex of Guam, pallidonigral degener-ation, Wilson's disease, and Huntington's disease.

This chapter will focus on the most relevant differential diagnoses of PD. We will examine those disorders with neurologic, neuropsychiatric, and neuropsychologic symptoms similar to PD, as well as the relevance of vascular lesions and exposure to neuroleptic drugs for the production of parkinsonian signs.

Table 3.1. Etiologic classification of parkinsonism (akinetic–rigid syndrome)

Idiopathic PD

Secondary parkinsonism ("Parkinson's plus")

A. *Other primary degenerative brain diseases*
• Olivopontocerebellar atrophies ⎫
• Shy–Drager syndrome   ⎬ multiple system atrophy
• Striatonigral degeneration   ⎭
• Progressive supranuclear palsy
• Parkinson-dementia-amyotrophic lateral sclerosis complex
• Alzheimer's disease
• Pick's disease
• Corticobasal ganglionic degeneration
• Corticostriatospinal degeneration
• Azorean disease
• Huntington's disease*
• Familial basal ganglionic calcification*
• Pallidal degenerations*
• Neuroacanthocytosis
• Hallervorden–Spatz disease*
• L-dopa-responsive dystonia-parkinsonism*
• Others* (e.g., familial depression, alveolar hypoventilation, and parkinsonism; X-linked
  Philippine dystonia-parkinsonism)

B. *Secondary parkinsonism due to other causes*
• Drugs* (dopamine receptor blockers, dopamine depletors, lithium, alpha-methyldopa)
• Toxins* (manganese, MPTP, mercury, methanol, ethanol, carbon disulfide)
• Anoxic encephalopathy* (including carbon monoxide, cyanide)
• Vascular (atherosclerotic, hypertensive, amyloid angiopathy, Binswanger's disease)
• Postencephalitic* (encephalitis lethargica, other viral encephalitis, Creutzfeldt–Jakob disease)
• Head injury*
• Brain tumor*
• Hydrocephalus*
• Metabolic diseases* (e.g., Wilson's disease, acquired hepatocerebral degeneration,
  hypoparathyroidism, GM_1 gangliosidosis, Gaucher's disease, mitochondrial pathologies)

*Disorders that may cause juvenile parkinsonism.

Table 3.2. "Red flags" suggestive of an atypical parkinsonian disorder

Lower body parkinsonism
Absent or atypical dyskinesias
Absent, poor, or waning responses to l-dopa
Autonomic failure
Blepharospasm
Cerebellar signs
Muscular spasms
Early-onset dementia
Disproportionate antecollis/retrocollis
Early-onset instability and falls
Early-onset or severe sialorrhea
Pathologic affective display
Eyelid apraxia (levator inhibition)
Marked frontal lobe syndrome (e.g., motor perseverations)
Fluctuating cognition and arousal
Ideomotor or ideatory apraxia
Inspiratory stridor/sighs
Myoclonus
Overstuffing mouth when eating
Early or severe speech and swallowing difficulties
Pyramidal signs
Rapid disease progression
Sensory or visual neglect/cortical sensory distribution
Snoring/restless sleep
Supranuclear gaze palsy/slowing of saccades
Very sparse blink rate
Visual hallucinations not due to drugs

Progressive supranuclear palsy

Clinical vignette

A 74-year-old man was brought to the Movement Disorders Clinic in a wheelchair by his family. One year earlier, the patient noticed progressive clumsiness while walking, rigidity in upper and lower limbs, and marked difficulty in rising from an armless chair and turning in bed. He was diagnosed with PD and l-dopa was started. There was moderate initial benefit, but the l-dopa efficacy progressively wore off, and dosage increments, up to 1 g, did not produce further motor improvement. Speech became progressively unintelligible and frequent choking occurred during eating; gait became very unsteady, and the patient had to use a wheelchair.

Clinical aspects

Progressive supranuclear palsy (PSP) is the neurodegenerative disorder most frequently misdiagnosed as PD (Agid et al., 1987; Golbe et al., 1988; Golbe, 1992). Litvan et al. (1996) proposed clinical criteria for this entity, which were reported to have a specificity of 100% and a sensitivity of 50% (Table 3.3). Initial symptoms of PSP are postural instability, supranuclear vertical gaze palsy, eyelid apraxia, bradykinesia, rigidity, and resting tremor. Rigidity is more axial than appendicular and tremor is less frequent than in PD. Dysarthria may appear about 2 years after the onset of motor symptoms, and dysphagia may begin between 1–2 years after the onset of dysarthria (Muller et al., 2001). Later symptoms of PSP are pseudobulbar palsy and dementia, and response to l-dopa is usually poor or absent. With disease progression, PSP patients are still able to keep relatively more erect than PD patients, sometimes with neck hyperextension and a tendency to fall backwards. The most frequent sign in patients with PSP is supranuclear gaze palsy, with marked limitation of vertical gaze (downward in particular). Pathologic laughing or crying (i.e., sudden emotional displays without an appropriate underlying emotional stimulus) is also frequent. A recent study, which compared the frequency of psychiatric disorders between 61 patients with PSP and 103 patients with PD, demonstrated significantly more severe apathy and disinhibition in PSP, and a significantly higher frequency of hallucinations, delusions, and depression in PD (Aarsland et al., 2001). PSP patients only rarely show asymmetric parkinsonism, unilateral dystonia, or apraxia (Table 3.4), but may develop greater cognitive impairments than patients with PD (Soliveri et al., 2000).

Laboratory findings

MRI studies in PSP reported moderate to severe atrophy of the midbrain and diencephalon, and thinning of the superior part of the quadrigeminal plate in more than 50% of patients (Savoiardo et al., 1994). Schultz et al. (1999) demonstrated that MRI volumetric measurements of the brainstem,

Table 3.3. Criteria for the clinical diagnosis of progressive supranuclear palsy (PSP)

Definite PSP
- Defined by histologic confirmation

Probable PSP
- Gradually progressive disorder
- Onset at age 40 years or later
- Vertical supranuclear ophthalmoparesis and prominent postural instability with falls within the first year of symptom onset

Possible PSP
- Gradually progressive disorder
- Onset at age 40 years or later, and either:
- Vertical supranuclear ophthalmoparesis
  or
- Slowing of vertical saccades and prominent postural instability with falls within the first year of symptom onset

Exclusion criteria for both probable and possible PSP
- Clinical findings compatible with encephalitis lethargica
- "Alien hand" syndrome, cortical sensory deficits, focal frontal or temporoparietal atrophy
- Hallucinations or delusions unrelated to dopaminergic therapy
- Cortical dementia of Alzheimer's type (severe amnesia, aphasia, or agnosia)
- Prominent cerebellar symptomatology or unexplained dysautonomia (early, or severe incontinence, impotence, or symptomatic postural hypotension)
- Severe asymmetry of parkinsonian signs
- Neuroradiologic evidence of relevant structural abnormalities (e.g., basal ganglia or brain stem infarcts, lobar atrophy)
- Whipple's disease, confirmed by polymerase chain reaction

Supportive features (not required for diagnosis)
- Symmetric akinesia or rigidity, proximal more than distal
- Retrocollis
- Poor, absent, or transient response of parkinsonism to l-dopa therapy
- Early dysarthria and dysphagia
- Early cognitive impairment, including at least two of the following: apathy, impaired abstract thought, decreased verbal fluency, or frontal "release" signs

Adapted from Litvan et al. (1996).

Table 3.4. PD and PSP: clues for clinical diagnosis

	PD	PSP
Postural stability	Early instability is rarely a feature of PD	Falls, often backward, are a frequent presenting feature
Positive l-dopa response	Always	Absent, poor, or waning
L-dopa-induced dyskinesias	Very frequent in advanced stages of the disease	Uncommon, but may develop dystonia late in the disease
Gaze abnormalities	Elderly patients with PD may have limitation of upgaze and convergence. Voluntary vertical saccades are normal.	Marked slowing and limitation of vertical gaze
Blink rate	Diminished	Severely diminished
Speech	Early or severe speech and swallowing difficulties do not suggest PD. Stuttering or palilalia may occur at a late stage in a minority of PD patients.	Frequent, low-pitched, "growling" dysarthria; Stuttering or palilalia may be an early feature of the disease
Sialorrhea	Rarely severe, usually a late sign	Profuse and early
Pyramidal signs	Not a feature of PD	Present in one-third of patients
Symmetry of parkinsonism	Asymmetric	Mostly symmetric
Posture	Flexed	Axial rigidity and disproportionate retrocollis
Pathologic affective display	Low frequency	High frequency
"Frontal lobe" signs	Mild and only present on specific testing	High frequency
Mean age at onset	60 years	63 years
Dysphagia	Rarely an early feature	Severe dysphagia is common

cerebellum, caudate nucleus, and putamen are useful in discriminating PD from both PSP and multiple system atrophy. Studies using [^{18}F] fluorodeoxyglucose positron emission tomography (^{18}FDG-PET) or iodo-amphetamine single photon emission computed tomography (SPECT) in PSP showed consistent blood flow reductions in the frontal lobes and striatum, but the sensitivity and specificity of these findings have not been established (D'Antona et al., 1985; Foster et al., 1988; Leenders et al., 1988; Blin et al., 1990; Brooks, 1994).

Neuropathologic findings

PSP is characterized by a high density of neurofibrillar tangles and neuropil threads in the globus pallidus, subthalamic nucleus, substantia nigra, and pons, and less frequent involvement of the striatum, oculomotor complex, medulla, and dentate nucleus (Hauw et al., 1994; Collins et al., 1995; Verny et al., 1996).

Multisystem atrophy

Clinical vignette

A 51-year-old man came to the Movement Disorders Clinic because of a 2-month history of progressive rigidity and slowness. He also reported increased salivation, severe constipation, and loss of sexual potency. Physical examination showed a mild akinetic–rigid syndrome and orthostatic hypotension. L-dopa treatment was started and doses were progressively increased up to 1 g per day, but parkinsonian signs remained unchanged and orthostatic hypotension worsened.

Clinical aspects

Multisystem atrophy (MSA) consists of a group of neurodegenerative disorders, including: striatonigral degeneration (Adams et al., 1964) whenever parkinsonism predominates, Shy–Drager syndrome (Shy & Drager, 1960) whenever autonomic failure predominates, and olivopontocerebellar atrophy (Dejerine & Thomas, 1900) whenever cerebellar features predominate (Table 3.5). Most patients with MSA show akinesia, which is mainly asymmetric, and tremor, which may be postural and/or resting. Autonomic dysfunction was reported to be present in 97% of patients, pyramidal features in 54%, cerebellar signs in 34%, and other signs, such as postural instability and cognitive impairment, in less than one-third of the patients (Soliveri et al., 2000) (Tables 3.6 and 3.7). Dysarthria and dysphagia usually develop about 2 years and 5 years after the onset of the disease, respectively (Muller et al., 2001).

Table 3.5. Subtypes of multisystem atrophy

	Parkinsonian signs	Pyramidal signs	Cerebellar signs	Autonomic dysfunction
Olivopontocerebellar atrophy	+	+	+++	+
Striatonigral degeneration	+++	+	–	+
Shy–Drager syndrome	+	+	–	+++

– Absent

+ Mild

+++ Severe

Table 3.6. Criteria for the clinical diagnosis of multisystem atrophy

Autonomic dysfunction (defined as a fall of 30 mmHg of systolic blood pressure and/or 15 mmHg of diastolic blood pressure or urinary incontinence or incomplete voiding plus impotence)

Parkinsonism (defined as bradykinesia plus one or more of the following: rigidity, postural instability, and postural or resting tremor)

Cerebellar dysfunction (defined as gait ataxia plus one or more of the following: ataxic dysarthria, limb ataxia, and evoked nystagmus)

Corticospinal dysfunction (e.g., extensor plantar response plus hyperreflexia)

Adapted from Gilman et al. (1999).

Laboratory findings

Autonomic tests such as the tilt test (which may demonstrate orthostatic hypotension and compensatory failure of cardiac reflexes) and anal sphincter electromyography (which may demonstrate marked neurogenic changes) were reported to be abnormal in more than 90% of patients (Colosimo et al., 1995; Magalhaes et al., 1995). MRI studies may show cerebellar or brain stem atrophy and hypointensities of the putamen (Olanow, 1992; Konagaya et al., 1994), but the specificity of these findings for the diagnosis of MSA is not known. PET studies using the D_2 receptor ligand, raclopride, demonstrated a significantly lower D_2 striate binding in MSA patients compared with patients with PD, and similar findings were reported using SPECT and the radioligand, [123I] idiobenzamide (van

Table 3.7. PD and MSA: clues for clinical diagnosis

	PD	MSA
Postural faintness	Rare in the absence of dopaminergic medication	Present in about 70% of patients
Incontinence	Gradual development of detrusor hyperreflexia, resulting in frequency and urgency	Frank incontinence and whole-bladder emptying are early features of the disease
Impotence	In older subjects	A frequent early problem
Pyramidal signs	Absent	Present in about 50% of patients
Positive response to l-dopa	Always	Mostly negative. Thirty percent of patients may show a short-lasting response.
L-dopa-induced dyskinesias	Frequent after 2 or 3 years of treatment	Atypical dyskinesias
Sweating	Common in l-dopa-treated patients	Excessive sweating followed by absent sweating
Cerebellar signs	Absent	Limb ataxia in about one-half, cerebellar gait ataxia in about one-third, and nystagmus in one-quarter of patients
Laryngeal stridor	Inspiratory stridor is rare	Inspiratory stridor in one-third of patients
Myoclonus	Absent	Myoclonic jerks of the fingers are present in one-third of patients
Pathologic affective display	Low frequency	High frequency
Swallowing difficulties	Late in the illness	Early and severe speech and swallowing difficulties
Speech	Hypophonic and monotone speech	Slurring cerebellar dysarthria, higher-pitched quivering, and strained or croaky speech
Symmetry of parkinsonism	Asymmetric	Symmetric

Royen et al., 1993). Friess et al. (2001) measured the growth hormone (GH) response to apomorphine in 16 patients with MSA, in 17 patients with PD, and in 11 healthy controls. They found a significantly greater GH response to apomorphine in patients with PD compared with patients with MSA or the control group, and suggested that the GH response to a subthreshold dose of apomorphine may be useful to identify patients with PD or MSA.

Neuropathologic findings

MSA is characterized by oligodendroglial argyrophilic cytoplasmic inclusions, neuronal loss, astrocytic gliosis, and pigment deposition in the striatum, substantia nigra, inferior olives, pons, cerebellum, and the intermediolateral cell columns of the spinal cord (Papp & Lantos, 1992; Lantos, 1995; Wenning et al., 1995).

Dementia with Lewy bodies

Clinical vignette

A 70-year-old retired lawyer was brought to the Neurology Clinic due to progressive physical and intellectual decline. His movements were slow, he had an expressionless face, and he reported increasing difficulties in turning in bed and rising from an armless chair. The main findings from neurologic examination were hypophonia, right-hand clumsiness, and mild resting tremor. His intellectual performance fluctuated during the day, with confusion and incoherence in the early afternoon and night-time. One night, he called the police, saying he could see "people talking in the balcony."

Clinical aspects

Dementia with Lewy bodies (DLB) is the second most common cause of dementia after Alzheimer's disease, and is characterized by fluctuating cognitive impairment, prominent attentional deficits, visuospatial dysfunction, visual hallucinations, and parkinsonian signs (McKeith et al., 2000). McKeith et al. (1996) proposed standardized criteria for probable and possible DLB, which include "core" and "supportive" features (Table 3.8).

Core features include progressive mental impairment and at least three of the following:

1 *Fluctuation in cognitive function* Deficits in cognitive performance may alternate with periods of normality or near normality, daytime

Table 3.8. Criteria for the clinical diagnosis of probable and possible dementia with Lewy bodies (DLB)

---

1. Progressive cognitive decline of sufficient magnitude to interfere with normal social or occupational function. Prominent or persistent memory impairment may not necessarily occur in the early stages but is usually evident with progression of the disease. Deficits on tests of attention, fronto-subcortical skills, and visuospatial ability may be prominent

2. Two of the following core features are necessary for a diagnosis of probable DLB, and one is necessary for a diagnosis of possible DLB:
   • Fluctuating cognition with pronounced variation in attention and alertness
   • Recurrent visual hallucinations that are typically well formed and detailed
   • Spontaneous motor features of parkinsonism

3. Features supportive of the diagnosis are:
   • Repeated falls
   • Syncope
   • Transient loss of consciousness
   • Neuroleptic sensitivity
   • Systematized delusions
   • Hallucinations in other modalities

4. A diagnosis of DLB is less likely in the presence of:
   • Strokes (e.g., positive neurologic signs, or vascular lesions on brain imaging)
   • Evidence on physical examination or laboratory investigation of any physical illness or other brain disorder that sufficiently accounts for the clinical picture

---

Adapted from McKeith et al. (2000).

drowsiness, or transient confusion. Keeping diaries of cognitive performance may be useful, and recent studies described reliable scales to rate fluctuations (Walker et al., 2000).

2 *Visual hallucinations* These phenomena are clinically similar to hallucinations arising from anticholinergic or other antiparkinsonian medication, or during delirium due to systemic illness. People or animals hidden behind room furniture or in a garden are the images most frequently reported (McKeith et al., 1996). Emotional responses to hallucinations are variable, and range from indifference and retained insight (i.e., hallucinosis) to lack of insight and belief in the reality of the false perception (i.e., true hallucinations) (Ballard et al., 1999).

3 *Motor parkinsonism* Rigidity and bradykinesia are the most frequent neurologic signs of DLB, but masked face, hypophonia, and flexed posture with shuffling gait are also common. Tremor is present in 2–55% of DLB patients. In a study with pathologic confirmation of the diagnosis, Ballard et al. (1997) reported that resting tremor, bradykinesia, action tremor, lack of facial expression, and rigidity were the most frequent neurologic signs in DLB. Louis et al. (1997) compared the prevalence of parkinsonian signs in patients with either DLB or PD and found resting tremor to be more frequent in PD (85%) than in DLB (55%), whereas myclonus was more frequent in DLB (19%) than in PD (0%). There were no significant between-group differences in the frequency of rigidity and bradykinesia, and a positive response to l-dopa was present in 100% of PD patients compared with 70% of DLB patients (Louis et al., 1997). Parkinsonism, myclonus, the absence of resting tremor, and a negative response to l-dopa have a positive predictive value for DLB of 85% (McKeith et al., 1996).

4 *Supportive features* Additional frequent findings in DLB are repeated falls, hypotonia, syncope, and transient loss of consciousness, which may be a severe manifestation of fluctuation in attention and cognition (McKeith et al., 1992). Treatment of confusional states with neuroleptics may produce increased mortality and morbidity. Initially, patients may show increased sedation and sudden onset of rigidity, postural instability, and falls, with progressive deterioration in cognitive performance, confusion, and fixed flexion posture followed by a significant decrease in liquid and food intake (Burke et al., 1998). Some patients may show tactile, olfactory, and auditory hallucinations, but these manifestations are not frequent.

In a retrospective study, which included 24 patients who underwent neuropathologic examination, Mega et al. (1996) reported a sensitivity of 75% and a specificity of 79% for the DLB criteria. More recent studies replicated the high specificity of these criteria (95–100%), but sensitivity ranged from 22% to 83% (Holmes et al., 1999; McKeith et al., 2000). Several studies examined the longitudinal evolution of DLB (e.g., Olichney et al., 1998) and found a significantly faster cognitive decline and higher mortality in DLB patients than in Alzheimer's disease (AD) patients.

Laboratory findings

There are no specific abnormalities on CT or MRI examination in DLB: patients may show generalized cortical atrophy or relatively more severe frontal lobe involvement. There is less medial temporal atrophy in DLB than in AD (Barber et al., 1999), and SPECT findings are similar to those reported in AD, usually with dorsal frontal and bilateral temporoparietal hypoperfusion (Talbot et al., 1998). However, a [123I] idioamphetamine SPECT study revealed relatively lower cerebral blood flow in the occipital lobes, and relatively higher right medial temporal cerebral blood flow, in DLB patients compared with AD patients (Ishii et al., 1999), whereas Hu et al. (2000), using the [18F] fluorodopa PET technique, described a significant reduction of striatal dopamine uptake in DLB patients compared with AD patients.

Neuropathologic findings

Whereas Lewy bodies are the core pathologic feature in clinically diagnosed DLB, there is also neuronal loss in the substantia nigra, locus coeruleus, dorsal nucleus of the vagus, hypothalamus, and forebrain cholinergic nuclei; spongiform changes may be found in the temporal lobes (Kosaka et al., 1984). Dickson et al. (1994) reported ubiquitin-positive dystrophic Lewy neurites in the hippocampus, and more than 20 different antigenic determinants such as synaptophysin have been identified in LBs. The importance of Alzheimer-type pathology in DLB remains controversial: β-Amyloid plaques are present in the cortex of most, but not all, cases of DLB, but neurofibrillar tangles are rare (Perry et al., 1990). Parkinsonian signs in DLB were reported to correlate with reduced dopamine concentration in the basal ganglia (Perry et al., 1997). The dopamine D_2 receptor upregulation in the basal ganglia typical of PD is absent in DLB (Piggott et al., 1999), and there is a significantly lower density of cortical cholinergic receptors compared with AD (Langlais et al., 1993).

Secondary parkinsonism

Parkinsonian signs may result from metabolic disorders and lesions to specific brain areas produced by cerebrovascular disease (so called "vascular parkinsonism"), head trauma, intoxication with drugs or heavy metals, hydrocephalus, brain tumors, infections, or Wilson's disease (Fahn, 1977) (Table 3.1). We will briefly address each of the most frequent causes of secondary parkinsonism.

Drug-induced parkinsonism
Clinical vignette

A 50-year-old woman visited a general practitioner complaining of painful stiffness in her arms and legs. Upon physical examination, the patient had poor bilateral arm swing and masked face. A tentative diagnosis of PD was made, and the patient was referred to a Movement Disorders Clinic. There was a history of cinnarizine intake due to dizziness for 9 months prior to the onset of physical symptoms, and physical examination demonstrated bradykinesia and flexed posture, but no resting tremor. The patient was given a single dose of 200/50 mg of l-dopa/carbidopa, without subsequent motor improvement, and cinnarizine was stopped. Three months later, the patient was greatly improved, with full remission of her parkinsonian signs 2 months later.

The prevalence of drug-induced parkinsonism (DIP) was reported to range between 15% and 40% (Fahn, 1977). Table 3.9 lists those drugs that most frequently produce parkinsonism (McLolland, 1978; Marti Masso et al., 1991). Parkinsonian signs usually improve weeks to a few months after withdrawing the causal agent, with complete remission after 6 months of drug withdrawal in most patients (Ayd, 1961; Owens et al., 1982). Anticholinergic drugs or amantadine may provide some benefit in patients who are not able to discontinue the causal drug. The efficacy of oral l-dopa in treating DIP was examined in small case series, and results have not been impressive (Bruno & Bruno, 1966; Mindham, 1976). Merello et al. (1996) examined the usefulness of l-dopa and apomorphine in treating DIP in a series of 12 patients with schizophrenia and chronic neuroleptic treatment, but neither drug produced a significant benefit.

Toxic and mood-related parkinsonism

Toxic agents, and metabolic agents such as manganese, carbon monoxide poisoning, and mercurials, may cause non-focal and symmetric parkinsonian signs, but focal or asymmetric parkinsonism does not rule out the diagnosis of secondary parkinsonism. Bradykinesia, rigidity, and postural abnormalities may be found in some psychiatric disorders such as depression and catatonia (Starkstein et al., 1996).

Table 3.9. Drugs associated with parkinsonism

Drugs most commonly reported to produce parkinsonism	Drugs sometimes reported to produce parkinsonism	Drugs with isolated reports of parkinsonism
Antidepressants	**Anticonvulsants**	**Oral contraceptives**
fluoxetine	phenytoin	Premarin
amoxapine	valproate	
phenelzine		
lithium		
Anti-emetics	**Antihistamines**	**Benzodiazepines**
prochilorperazine	cimetidine	diazepam
metoclopramide		
remoxipride		
sulpiride		
Neuroleptics		**Miscellaneous**
phenothiazines		captopril
butyrophenones		pindolol
thioxanthenes		procaine
dibenzoxazepines		amiodarone
		vincristine
		cytosine arabinoside
		meperidine
		alfa-methyldopa
		disulfiram
		bethanechol
		anti-inflammatory agents
Catecholamine-depleting agents		**Antimicrobials**
reserpine		cephaloridine
tetrabenazine		trimethoprim
alpha-methyltyrosine		sulfamethoxazole
Calcium channel blockers		
cinnarizine		
flunarizine		
diltiazem		

Clinical vignette

J.M. was a 50-year-old surgeon who came to the office complaining of bilateral hand tremor and motor slowness. He had a major depressive episode 2 years before, which lasted for 5 months and remitted spontaneously. Six months later, he had a recurrence of depression together with gait instability and frequent falls. On physical examination, J.M. had mild bilateral tremor on both hands, mild rigidity and bradykinesia in the upper limbs, gait slowness, and mild postural instability. He cried during the interview, and worried about being unable to continue his work as a surgeon due to his tremor. He had severe insomnia, poor appetite with marked weight loss, loss of interest in hobbies, loss of libido, and marked anxiety. A diagnosis of major depression was made, and the patient was started on nortriptyline (80 mg per day). Six weeks later, the patient had a full remission of his major depressive episode, and reported only mild early insomnia. Physical examination showed a marked recovery of the motor signs: there was no tremor, movements were wide and brisk, and gait, posture, and stability were all normal.

In 1921, Kraepelin had already reported that depressed patients may show "movements . . . carried out with . . . reduced speed and without vigor," and that "behavior is still . . . expression rigid and immobile." Both bradyphrenia and bradykinesia have been consistently reported in subgroups of depressed patients. Starkstein et al. (2001) reported that 20% of a series of 94 patients with "primary" (i.e., no known brain injury) depression had parkinsonism, defined as: "the presence of tremor and/or rigidity and bradykinesia." There was a significant correlation between the severity of parkinsonism and older age, more severe cognitive deficits, and more severe depression. An important finding of that study was that depressed patients with full remission of depression at follow-up showed a significant decrease in UPDRS (Unified Parkinson's Disease Rating Scale) scores, suggesting that parkinsonism in depression may be reversible upon the improvement of the mood disorder. On the other hand, depressed patients without remission of depression showed no improvement of parkinsonian signs and further cognitive decline, suggesting an underlying dementia disorder.

Vascular parkinsonism
Clinical vignette

A 68-year-old man with a history of heavy smoking, hypertension, and hypercholesterolemia had an ischemic heart attack treated with angioplasty 10 years before the evaluation. After surgery, he developed progressive slowness and walking difficulties. At the evaluation, there was symmetric rigidity and bradykinesia involving primarily the

Table 3.10. Criteria for the clinical diagnosis of vascular parkinsonism

Vascular parkinsonism is diagnosed whenever patients have Parkinsonism (defined as the presence of a least two of the four cardinal symptoms of tremor at rest, bradykinesia, rigidity, and abnormal postural reflexes), and a score of 2 or more on the composite vascular score.

	Composite vascular score
Pathologically or angiographically proven vascular disease	2 points
Onset of parkinsonism within 1 month of a clinical stroke	1 point
History of two or more strokes	1 point
History of two or more risk factors for stroke	1 point
Neuroimaging evidence of vascular disease in two different arterial places	1 point

Adapted from Winikates & Jankovic (1999).

lower limbs, shuffling gait, freezing, and short steps. Rigidity in the lower limbs became worse during simultaneous movements of the upper limbs. The trunk was flexed and arm swing was present but reduced in amplitude. Reflexes were brisk with bilateral extensor plantar responses. An MRI scan showed severe, widespread, white matter hyperintensities with multiple lacunar infarcts.

Vascular lesions to the basal ganglia may produce parkinsonian signs that respond poorly to l-dopa therapy (Tolosa & Santamaria, 1984). There is usually lower body parkinsonism and gait abnormalities, but tremor is infrequent (Ikeda et al., 1996). Patients with multiple deep cerebral infarcts and white matter hyperintensities may show shuffling gait with preserved arm swing, a pattern known as "lower half" or "lower body" parkinsonism (Reider-Grosswasser et al., 1995). A history of strokes, heart disease, hypertension, and other risk factors for vascular disease further supports a diagnosis of vascular parkinsonism (Table 3.10) (Winikates & Jankovic, 1999). MRI scans in patients with acute-onset vascular parkinsonism may show vascular lesions in the subcortical gray nuclei (striatum, globus pallidus, and thalamus) and white matter areas (Zijlmans et al., 1995).

Corticobasal ganglionic degeneration

Clinical vignette

A 69-year-old man reported a progressive, painful rigidity of the right arm, and clumsiness in activities of daily living. He also noted that his right hand and forearm sometimes

Table 3.11. Criteria for the clinical diagnosis of corticobasal degeneration

Inclusion criteria

1. Chronic progressive course
2. Asymmetric at onset
3. Presence of cortical dysfunction, including:
   - ideomotor apraxia
   - cortical sensory loss
   - "alien limb" syndrome
4. Presence of a movement disorder, including an akinetic-rigid syndrome resistant to l-dopa, and either:
   - dystonic limb posturing
   - spontaneous reflex focal myoclonus
5. Presence of DSM-IV diagnostic criteria for dementia

Exclusion criteria

1. Presence of l-dopa responsivity (other than mild worsening on withdrawal)
2. Presence of typical parkinsonian resting tremor
3. Presence of severe autonomic disturbances, including symptomatic postural hypotension, urinary or bowel incontinence, and constipation to the point of repeated impaction
4. Presentation with cognitive disturbances (other than apraxia, or speech and language disorders)

Adapted from Litvan et al. (1997).

adopted abnormal postures, which affected his writing. On examination, he presented rigidity and bradykinesia restricted to the right upper limb, myoclonic jerks on the right hand, and asymmetric and brisk reflexes with plantar extension. L-dopa was started but there was no clinical improvement after 1 month of treatment. The disease rapidly progressed and the patient developed severe postural instability and gait disturbance. Two years after disease onset, the patient developed speech problems and severe swallowing impairment.

Clinical aspects

Corticobasal degeneration is a rare disorder described by Rebeiz et al. in 1968. The most frequent initial symptoms are unilateral clumsiness, cortical sensory loss, paresthesias, rigidity, and dysarthria (Gibb et al., 1991; Lang, 1992) (Table 3.11). Patients may show a dystonic posture of the affected limbs, ideomotor apraxia (i.e., a disturbance in programming the timing, sequencing, and spatial organization of gestural movements), and myclonus (Leiguarda et al., 1994; Brundt et al., 1995). Less than half of the patients may show the so-called "alien limb," characterized by wandering movements of the arm, which may interfere with purposeful movements. Gait disturbance and loss of postural reflexes are frequent findings, and falling backwards, dysarthria and dysphagia, supranuclear gaze abnormalities with upgaze limitation, and hypometric and slow saccades are present early in the disease (Gibb et al., 1989; Riley et al., 1990). Blinking abnormalities and blepharospasm are also frequent, and some patients may show early cognitive deficits (Pillon et al., 1996).

Laboratory studies

MRI scans usually show cortical atrophy in frontal and posterior parietal areas, mainly contralateral to the most affected side, as well as striatal hypointensities on T2-weighted images (Savoiardo et al., 1994; Grisoli et al., 1995; Hauser et al., 1996). PET studies using [18F] fluorodeoxyglucose usually show asymmetric hypometabolism in frontal and parietal regions (Sawle et al., 1991; Blin et al., 1992; Brooks, 1996).

Neuropathology

There is usually asymmetric cortical atrophy (mainly frontoparietal), cortical neuronal loss with astrocytic gliosis, vacuolized cortical neurons with poor staining ("neuronal achromasia"), and cytoplasmic hyalinization with vacuolization (Revesz et al., 1995). Loss of pigmented neurons in the substantia nigra is also frequent, but there are no Lewy bodies (Feany et al., 1996).

Alzheimer's disease

Clinical vignette

A 72-year-old woman with a 4-year history of dementia slowly developed shuffling gait, masked face, and poor arm swing. Upon physical examination, the patient had bilateral rigidity and bradykinesia, but no tremor. Treatment with l-dopa only produced a mild and short-lasting motor improvement.

Alzheimer's disease (AD) is a chronic disorder with progressive cognitive decline, and a prevalence of 2–4% in the population aged over 65 years.

Table 3.12. Dementia and parkinsonism: clues for clinical diagnosis

	PD with dementia	Dementia with Lewy bodies	Alzheimer's disease with parkinsonism
Initial symptoms	Parkinsonism	Parkinsonism, visual hallucinations, and cognitive fluctuations	Cognitive deficits
Onset of cognitive decline	Late	Early	Initial
Psychiatric symptoms	Late, and mainly related to medication	Early	Frequent, but with variable onset
Severity of parkinsonism	Severe, requires l-dopa treatment	Moderate severity; half of cases may require l-dopa therapy	Mild to moderate
Response to l-dopa	100%	70%	0%
Rest tremor	Very frequent (±85%)	Moderately frequent (±55%)	Rarely present
Myoclonus	Never	20% of cases	About one-third of cases
Rigidity and bradykinesia	Always	Always	Frequent
Dystonia	Frequent	Not reported	Not reported
Response to neuroleptics	Worsening of parkinsonism	Severe worsening of parkinsonism and behavior	Worsening of parkinsonism

Motor disturbances in AD include apraxia, myoclonus, gait disorders, and parkinsonian signs (Chen et al., 1991; Merello et al., 1994). Molsa et al. (1984) examined 143 patients with probable AD for the presence of parkinsonism and found that only 8% of them had no parkinsonian signs. In a more recent community-based study, Funkenstein (1993) demonstrated that diminished spontaneous movements of the limbs or face, reduced arm swing during walking, and gait abnormalities were associated with a substantially increased probability of having clinically diagnosed AD.

Based on findings of the Unified Parkinson's Disease Rating Scale (UPDRS), Merello et al. (1994) reported that 18 (23%) of a series of 78 AD patients met criteria for parkinsonism, and 44 (56%) had isolated parkinsonian signs (Table 3.12).

The mechanism of parkinsonism in AD is poorly understood. Whereas some studies demonstrated neuropathologic similarities between PD and AD with parkinsonism, other studies showed no abnormality of the nigrostriatal dopaminergic terminals in AD (Ditter & Mirra, 1987).

General conclusions

Standardized diagnostic criteria for PD, such as the UK PD Society's Brain Bank clinical criteria, were found to have high sensitivity but a relatively low specificity for PD. Disorders most often confused with PD are progressive supranuclear palsy and multisystem atrophy, followed by dementia with Lewy bodies, drug-induced and vascular parkinsonism, mood disorders, AD, and corticobasal degeneration. Non-PD parkinsonism is characterized by an akinetic–rigid syndrome and additional symptoms atypical of PD (e.g., blepharospasm, autonomic failure, cerebellar signs, ophthalmoparesis, severe cognitive fluctuations, unilateral apraxia, and pyramidal signs), as well as by a poor and short-lasting response to l-dopa or dopaminergic agonists. Drug-induced and vascular parkinsonism should be readily diagnosed, since parkinsonian signs may either improve or stabilize following the discontinuation of the causative drug or the treatment of vascular risk factors. Laboratory findings may help in the differential diagnosis of some of the disorders (e.g., vascular brain lesions in vascular parkinsonism, dysautonomia in multisystem atrophy, sphincter electromyography in progressive supranuclear palsy), but findings on physical examination and response to l-dopa remain the most useful diagnostic tools.

Cognitive deficits in Parkinson's disease

The French neurologist Charcot (1875) was the first to suggest the presence of intellectual deficits in PD, when he noticed that ". . . psychic faculties are definitely impaired . . . at a given point, the mind becomes clouded and the memory is lost." Since then, literally hundreds of studies have been devoted to examining the frequency and type of cognitive deficits in PD.

This chapter will review the prevalence of cognitive deficits and dementia in PD. We will examine the clinical correlates and potential mechanisms of cognitive impairments in PD, and neuropathologic findings in PD patients with dementia. The chapter is divided into two main sections: one devoted to dementia *sensu stricto*, and another devoted to deficits in specific cognitive domains. This separation does not mean that the above are independent phenomena, but allows a more coherent discussion of these topics.

Dementia in PD

Clinical vignette

J.B. is a 59-year-old lawyer, who came to the neurology clinic complaining of right-side stiffness and intermittent hand tremor. On physical examination he had mild right bradykinesia and cogwheel rigidity, and mild pill-rolling tremor. He agreed to participate in a research project, which included a comprehensive neuropsychologic evaluation. He showed no cognitive deficits, except for mild deficits on a verbal fluency task. At a follow-up evaluation 5 years later, he showed more severe bradykinesia and rigidity, which were bilateral but more severe on the right side. Tremor had increased, and he could only write with difficulty. He complained about not being as efficient as usual. He was unable to work with different problems simultaneously and could only concentrate on one thing at a time. On neuropsychologic evaluation there were mild deficits on a variety of cognitive tasks, primarily those tapping executive functions. Three years later, the patient showed a clear progression of parkinsonism, complaining of severe motor fluctuations and dystonic movements. He also had a progressive memory decline, and was no longer able to work as a lawyer. His wife stressed that he was unable to balance his check-book, and made errors in handling money. He was less interested in participating in social activities and usual hobbies. Neuropsychologic examination showed a Mini-Mental State Exam (MMSE) score of 21, and widespread deficits on most cognitive tasks.

Diagnosis of dementia

The first important issue is how to diagnose dementia in patients with a chronic neurologic condition, such as PD. Mindham (1999) stressed that PD patients fulfilling clinical criteria for dementia in PD may diverge in terms of clinical, psychometric, social, and behavioral measures, and warned that these subjects may suffer from a range of different cognitive disorders. Another limitation to the diagnosis of dementia in PD is the low level of agreement in the estimates of dementia provided by different classification systems. In a recent study, Erkinjuntti et al. (1997) examined the effects of six well-known classification systems: Diagnostic and Statistical Manual (DSM) III, III-R, and IV (American Psychiatric Association, 1994), International Classification of Diseases (ICD) 9 and 10 (World Health Organization, 1992), and the Cambridge Examination for Mental Disorders of the elderly (CAMDEX) (Roth et al., 1988). Based on these systems, they calculated the prevalence of dementia in a series of about 2000 individuals aged 65 years or older enrolled in the Canadian Study of Health and Aging. Prevalences of dementia ranged from 3.1%, using the ICD-10 criteria, to 29.1% when using the DSM-III criteria. This approximately ten-fold difference in the prevalence of dementia, depending on the criteria used for diagnosis, may have a serious impact on the estimation of the prevalence of dementia in PD, given the heterogeneity of the criteria that have been used for this purpose.

The DSM-IV is one of the few classification systems that provides specific clinical criteria for the diagnosis of dementia in PD (Table 4.1), although several limitations of this diagnostic scheme deserve further discussion. First, the DSM-IV states that dementia should be a direct consequence of PD, but there are no specific guidelines as to how to make this judgment

Table 4.1. DSM clinical criteria for dementia due to PD

A. The diagnosis requires the development of multiple cognitive deficits manifested by both:
   (1) memory impairment, and
   (2) one (or more) of the following cognitive disturbances:
      • aphasia
      • apraxia
      • agnosia
      • disturbance in executive functioning
B. The cognitive deficits cause significant impairment in social or occupational functioning and
   represent a significant decline from a previous level of functioning. Dementia is
   characterized by cognitive and motor slowing, executive dysfunction, and impairment in
   memory retrieval. Declining cognitive performance in patients with PD is frequently
   exacerbated by depression.

Adapted from DSM-IV.

(e.g., it is difficult to ascertain on clinical grounds whether cognitive deficits are a pathophysiologic consequence of PD or, for instance, a comorbid Alzheimer's disease (AD)). Second, the DSM-IV considers dementia associated with PD to be characterized by cognitive and motor slowing, executive dysfunction, and impairment in memory retrieval. However, this syndrome may not be specific to PD-dementia, since significant motor slowing may also be present in AD patients with parkinsonism, and neither cognitive slowing, nor executive dysfunction, nor impairment in memory retrieval may reliably separate PD-demented patients from patients with other dementias. The ICD-10 provides criteria for dementia in PD, which are illustrated in Table 4.2.

In conclusion, different diagnostic schemes have been proposed for the diagnosis of dementia in PD, but the ultimate validity of these strategies still remains to be empirically established.

Prevalence of dementia

The prevalence of dementia in PD was estimated to range from 20% to 40% (Marttila & Rinne, 1976; Brown & Marsden, 1984; Marder et al., 1995; Tison et al., 1995). This wide variability may depend on several factors, such as:

1 *the assessment methodology* – higher prevalences were reported in studies using comprehensive neuropsychologic instruments compared with

Table 4.2. ICD clinical criteria for dementia due to PD

A. There is evidence of each of the following:
  (1) A decline in memory, which is most evident in the learning of new information although, in more severe cases, the recall of previously learned information may also be affected. The severity of the decline, with mild impairment as the threshold for diagnosis, should be assessed as follows:

  Mild: the degree of memory loss is sufficient to interfere with everyday activities, though not so severe as to be incompatible with independent living.

  Moderate: the degree of memory loss represents a serious handicap to independent living.

  Severe: the degree of memory loss is characterized by the complete inability to retain new information.

  (2) A decline in other cognitive abilities characterized by deterioration in judgment and thinking, such as planning and organizing, and in the general processing of information.

B. Awareness of the environment is preserved during a period of time that is sufficiently long as to allow the unequivocal demonstration of the symptoms in criterion A. When there are superimposed episodes of delirium, the diagnosis of dementia should be deferred.

C. There is a decline in emotional control or motivation, or a change in social behavior manifested as at least one of the following:
  • emotional lability
  • irritability
  • apathy
  • coarsening of social behavior

D. For a confident clinical diagnosis, the symptoms in criterion A should have been present for at least 6 months; if the period since the onset of symptoms is shorter, the diagnosis can be only tentative.

E. A diagnosis of PD has been established.

F. None of the cognitive impairment is attributable to antiparkinsonian medication.

G. There is no evidence of other causes of dementia.

Adapted from ICD-10.

studies using screenings of global cognitive function. For instance, Hobson and Meara (1999) demonstrated that the cognitive section of the Cambridge Examination for Mental Disorders (CAMCOG) was more sensitive than the MMSE in detecting cognitive impairment;

2 *the proportion of patients with early vs late onset of parkinsonian symptoms* – the prevalence of dementia was found to be higher in patients with a late onset of illness (Mohr et al., 1995);

3 *the definition of dementia* – i.e., whether dementia was diagnosed based
on standardized vs. "ad-hoc" criteria (Erkinjuntti et al., 1997);
4 *the severity of motor impairment* – the prevalence of dementia was reported to increase along the stages of the illness (0% in Hoehn & Yahr
stage I, 6% in stage II, 16% in stage III, 35% in stage IV, and 57% in stage
V (Growdon et al., 1990)).

Phenomenology of dementia

Cummings and Benson (1984) separated the dementias into cortical types
(e.g., AD) and subcortical types (e.g., PD, Huntington's disease) based on
the presence of qualitative differences in cognitive, emotional, and motor
impairments. In cortical dementias, cognitive deficits were reported to
include impairments in language and memory, agnosia, and apraxia,
whereas subcortical dementias were considered to be associated with a
relatively greater general slowness of thought processes and impaired ma-
nipulation of acquired knowledge, such as deficits in abstracting abilities,
retrieval of information, and visuospatial functions. Emotional disturbances in cortical dementias were characterized by a lack of awareness of
cognitive deficits and disinhibited behaviors, whereas subcortical dementias
were characterized by a higher prevalence of apathy and depression. Finally,
whereas motor deficits were reported to be absent in cortical dementias,
disorders of movement, tone, posture, and gait are prominent findings in
subcortical dementias.

We will now review relevant studies on the cognitive, emotional and
motor differential impairments in cortical and subcortical dementias, and
illustrate the phenomenology of dementia in PD.

Cognitive differences between cortical and subcortical dementias

Most studies using screening measures of global cognitive performance
found no significant differences between patients with cortical or subcortical dementias, whereas studies using more comprehensive neuropsychologic measures were able to demonstrate some significant between-
group differences (see Mohr et al., 1995, for a comprehensive review).
Cummings et al. (1988) compared AD patients and PD-demented patients
with similar global cognitive deficits on a series of speech and language
tasks. AD patients had more severe anomia and less information content in

spontaneous speech, whereas patients with PD-dementia had more gram-
matically simplified utterances and dysarthria. Both Litvan et al. (1991) and
Pillon et al. (1986) reported more severe deficits in executive functions in
patients with PD-dementia, whereas AD patients had more severe deficits
on delayed recall tasks of episodic memory (i.e., memory for past events). In
a study in which PD-demented patients were matched with a group of AD
patients for overall dementia severity, both groups had a similar performance on visuospatial tasks that were independent of memory function, but
PD-demented patients performed significantly worse than AD patients on
memory-dependent visuospatial tasks (Mohr et al., 1990a). Finally, Pate
and Margolin (1994) demonstrated that PD-demented patients had significantly more severe cognitive slowing (as measured with a reaction time
task) than a group of AD patients with a similar severity of overall cognitive
decline.

Other studies, however, could not find significant differences on memory
tasks between AD and PD-dementia. Leplow et al. (1997) reported no
significant differences on a test of remote memory for public events between
14 PD-demented patients and 16 patients with AD or vascular dementia
with a comparable degree of cognitive deficits. Kuzis et al. (1999) assessed
the differential impairment of explicit memory (i.e., the direct and conscious recollection of facts or information from previous learning episodes)
and implicit memory (i.e., the non-conscious remembering expressed
through improved performance of specific operations comprising a particular task with previous exposure) in a study that included 15 patients
with AD, 10 PD-demented patients, 15 non-demented PD patients, and 24
age-comparable normal controls. Patients and controls were all assessed
with tests of explicit memory (Buschke Selective Reminding Test, Benton
Visual Retention Test, and Digit Span) and tests of implicit memory
(Word-stem Completion Task and the Maze Test). The main finding was
that both AD and PD-dementia groups showed similar deficits on all
measures of explicit memory, and performed significantly worse than PD
patients without dementia, or controls. On the other hand, there were no
significant differences in any of the measures of implicit memory between
demented and non-demented groups. Starkstein et al. (1996) assessed 33
PD-demented patients and 33 patients with AD matched for age, sex, and
MMSE scores with a comprehensive neuropsychological assessment that

included tests of verbal memory, visual memory, auditory attention, concept formation and set shifting, verbal fluency, and visuospatial reasoning. They found that PD-demented patients had significantly lower scores than AD patients on a test of visuospatial reasoning (Raven's Progressive Matrices). Similar findings were reported by Sahakian et al. (1988), who found that patients with PD-dementia performed significantly worse than patients with AD on tests of visual discrimination learning and attentional set-shifting. On the other hand, Starkstein et al. (1996) could not find significant differences between AD and PD-dementia patients on other cognitive functions, suggesting that differential impairments in cognitive abilities in cortical vs subcortical dementias are not widespread and may be restricted to a few cognitive domains.

One factor that may help to explain some of the discrepant findings in the cognitive profile of cortical and subcortical dementias is the presence of heterogeneity in the cognitive deficits of PD-dementia. Mohr et al. (1995) described subgroups of PD patients with different profiles of cognitive deficits: one group had severe cognitive impairments and homogeneous deficits across cognitive domains, a second group had prominent deficits on visuospatial skills and relative preservation of executive functions, and a third group had relatively more severe deficits on executive functions and less impairments on visuospatial skills.

Few studies examined longitudinal changes in cognitive functions in cortical vs subcortical dementias. Stern et al. (1998) carried out a prospective comparative study of the evolution of 40 AD and 40 PD-demented patients matched for age, years of follow-up, and years of education. They found a similar rate of cognitive decline in a series of neuropsychologic tasks that assessed general cognition, verbal fluency, and abstract thinking for both groups, but PD-demented patients showed a significantly greater decline than the AD group on tasks of naming and verbal memory.

Emotional differences between cortical and subcortical dementias

Several studies examined the prevalence of affective changes in cortical dementias (primarily AD) and found a relatively high prevalence of both depression (about 20–40%) (Migliorelli et al., 1995) and apathy (about 20%) (Starkstein et al., 1995). On the other hand, few studies examined the prevalence of emotional problems among patients with subcortical

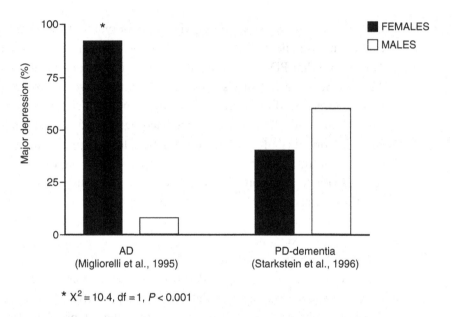

Figure 4.1. Major depression in PD-dementia was found to be more prevalent in males, whereas major depression in Alzheimer's disease (AD) was found to be more prevalent in females.

dementias. In their study comparing 33 AD patients with 33 PD-demented patients matched for age, gender, and global cognitive deficits, Starkstein et al. (1996) found that patients with PD and dementia had a significantly higher prevalence of major depression than patients with AD. This difference was gender-related, since major depression in PD-dementia was more prevalent in males, whereas major depression in AD was reported to occur significantly more often among females (Migliorelli et al., 1995) (Figure 4.1). Thus, differences in the prevalence of major depression between cortical and subcortical dementias may be related to the proportion of male and female patients in each group. Another finding in Starkstein et al.'s (1996) study was that anosognosia (i.e., unawareness of cognitive impairments) and disinhibition were both more severe in AD patients than in PD-demented patients, but no significant between-group differences were found in scores of apathy, irritability, and delusions.

Motor differences in cortical and subcortical dementias

Whereas parkinsonian signs such as tremor, rigidity, bradykinesia, and postural instability are the hallmark of PD, the proportion of these signs is quite variable, and several authors proposed subgroups of PD such as tremor-dominant or akinetic–rigid forms (e.g., Zetusky et al., 1985; Jankovic et al., 1990). The akinetic–rigid variant was reported to be associated with a significantly higher prevalence of dementia than the tremor-dominant or classical variant (Mayeux et al., 1981; Ebmeier et al., 1990), but this association could not always be confirmed (Paulus & Jellinger, 1991).

Parkinsonian signs were also reported to occur in patients with cortical dementias as well as among elderly individuals without cognitive or overt physical impairments. Ellis et al. (1996) suggested that parkinsonian signs may be a preclinical manifestation of AD, based on the finding that these signs may predict late-life dementia (Funkenstein et al., 1993), and that elderly individuals with isolated cognitive impairment are more likely to develop overt dementia if parkinsonian signs are present initially (Richards et al., 1993). The prevalence of parkinsonian signs in AD was reported to range between 6% and 50% (Lopez et al., 1997). This wide discrepancy may result from the inclusion in some studies of patients on neuroleptics, from different methodologies used to assess parkinsonism (e.g., studies using structured assessment scales produced higher rates of parkinsonism than studies using a routine clinical examination), and from differences in the relative severity of dementia (parkinsonian signs may become more severe in late stages of AD). The most frequent parkinsonian signs reported in AD are rigidity, bradykinesia, and facial masking, whereas resting tremor, On–Off fluctuations, and hypophonia are less frequent (Merello et al., 1994). Ellis et al. (1996) reported that 21% of a large series of community-dwelling neuroleptic-naive AD patients had parkinsonism, and during a 3-year follow-up period there was a 2–3% rate of incident bradykinesia, rigidity, and facial masking. Merello et al. (1994) assessed a consecutive series of 78 neuroleptic-naive patients with AD and 20 age-comparable normal controls using the Unified Parkinson's Disease Rating Scale (Fahn & Elton, 1987), and found that the prevalence of parkinsonism (defined as rigidity, bradykinesia, and/or resting tremor) was significantly higher in AD compared with normal controls (23% vs 0%, respectively). On the other hand, there were no significant between-group differences in the prevalence of isolated parkinsonian signs (defined as signs other than bradykinesia, rigidity, or resting tremor) (56% vs 57%, respectively).

Parkinsonian signs in AD may be a marker of a more aggressive dementing illness, since several studies demonstrated accelerated cognitive decline, shorter survival times, and poorer overall prognosis in AD patients with parkinsonism compared with those without parkinsonian signs (Stern et al., 1987; Chui et al., 1994). The question then arises as to whether the mechanism of parkinsonism in AD and PD is similar. Several findings argue against this hypothesis. First, significant cognitive deficits are a late finding in PD, whereas in AD parkinsonian signs usually develop concomitant to, or after, the onset of cognitive deficits (Merello et al., 1994). Second, for the two diseases to occur independently, the prevalence of both disorders among individuals aged 75–84 years should be about 0.25%, whereas the true prevalence of AD-parkinsonism is about 10 times higher (Ellis et al., 1996). Finally, whereas all the PD-demented patients in Starkstein et al.'s (1996) study had a positive response to l-dopa, AD patients with parkinsonism were reported not to improve upon treatment with dopaminergic agonists (Duret et al., 1989; Merello et al., 1994). Thus, other mechanisms besides concomitant PD were suggested to account for parkinsonism in AD, such as the presence of neurofibrillary tangles and neuropil threads in the substantia nigra (Liu et al., 1997), reduced substantia nigra neuron density (Kazee et al., 1995), reduced striatal dopamine activity (Langlais et al., 1993), loss of dopamine transporter sites in the nucleus accumbens, rostral caudate, and putamen (Murray et al., 1995), and the potential inclusion of patients with diffuse Lewy bodies in AD samples (Ellis et al., 1996).

Neuroimaging differences between cortical and subcortical dementias

Laasko et al. (1996) compared hippocampal volumes, as assessed through MRI, in a series of 50 patients with mild to moderate AD, 9 patients with vascular dementia, 12 PD patients without dementia, 8 PD patients with dementia, and 34 age-comparable normal controls. The main finding was that patients with either AD or PD-dementia had a comparable magnitude of hippocampal atrophy.

Starkstein et al. (1997) examined, with SPECT and [Tc 99m] hexamethylpropylene-amine oxime, a series of 18 non-demented PD patients, 12 demented PD patients, 24 AD patients, and 14 age-comparable normal

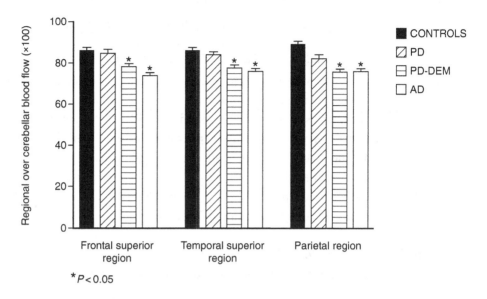

Figure 4.2. Patients with either Alzheimer's disease (AD) or PD-dementia (PD-DEM) had significantly bilateral hypoperfusion in superior temporal and parietal regions compared with non-demented PD patients and age-comparable healthy controls (*$P < 0.01$).

controls. The main finding was that patients with either AD or PD-dementia had significantly bilateral hypoperfusion in superior temporal, and parietal, regions compared with non-demented PD patients and normal controls (Figure 4.2). On the other hand, there were no significant differences in perfusion in any brain region between patients with AD or PD-dementia.

Van der Borgh et al. (1997) assessed with [18]FDG-PET a series of 9 AD patients, 9 PD-demented patients, and 9 normal controls. Both dementia groups were matched for gender, age, and general dementia severity. The main finding was that both AD and PD-dementia had a similar profile of metabolic deficits, with significant hypometabolism in parietal, temporal, frontal and posterior cingulate cortices compared with normal controls. The only between-group difference was that the PD-dementia group had less metabolic activity in the visual cortex but more metabolic activity in the medial temporal cortex compared with the AD group.

In conclusion, whereas there are no valid and reliable criteria to diagnose dementia in PD, several studies demonstrated some clinical differences between PD-dementia and AD. Patients with PD-dementia were reported to have more severe deficits on neuropsychologic tasks that assessed executive functions, visuospatial reasoning, visual discrimination learning, and set-shifting, whereas AD patients were reported to have more severe deficits on tasks that assessed naming, and both semantic and episodic memory, but these findings were not always confirmed. PD-demented patients were also reported to have a higher frequency of depression, whereas AD patients may show more severe anosognosia and disinhibition. However, parkinsonian signs, which are the hallmark of PD, were reported to be present in about 20–30% of AD patients, and neuroimaging studies comparing AD with PD-dementia produced mostly negative findings.

Clinical correlates of dementia

Duration of illness is one of the main clinical correlates of dementia in PD. In a 4-year longitudinal study, Biggins et al. (1992) found that 6% of a series of 87 patients with PD met DSM-III-R criteria for dementia at the initial evaluation. About 4 years later, the cumulative incidence of dementia among the PD sample was 19%, compared with none of a series of 50 normal control individuals with a similar length of follow-up. Biggins et al. (1992) further reported that those PD patients who became demented were older, had a longer duration of illness, and were older at onset of parkinsonian signs compared with those PD patients who did not become demented. Bayles et al. (1996) examined changes in MMSE scores in a group of 77 patients with PD and 43 normal controls during a 2-year follow-up period. They found that 22% of the PD patients had a 4-point decrement in MMSE scores at the time of follow-up, compared with none of the normal controls. Hughes et al. (2000) followed a cohort of 83 non-demented PD patients and 50 normal controls over a 10-year period and found a cumulative incidence of dementia in the PD group of 20%, compared with none in the control group. They found that age at entry into the study and severity of motor symptoms were significant predictors of dementia in PD. Hayashi et al. (1996) examined changes in motor function, cognition, and event-related potentials in 11 PD patients in Hoehn and Yahr stage II and 18 patients in stage III during a 2-year follow-up period. They found no significant changes in either ERPs or cognitive functions among those patients who had no change in motor functions during follow-up, but those who changed from stage III to stage IV (i.e., those who developed more severe motor symptoms over time) showed significant changes in ERPs and significant declines in scores of orientation, verbal recall, and constructional ability compared with patients who stayed within the same Hoehn and Yahr stage.

In a longitudinal study of newly diagnosed PD patients, Reid (1992) found that age at onset of parkinsonism and duration of illness were both important predictors of dementia: the prevalence of dementia was 8% in patients with an "early" onset of PD (<70 years) but 32% in those with a "late" onset (>70 years). At 3-year follow-up, prevalences of dementia were 18% and 83%, respectively. Caparros-Lefebvre et al. (1995) assessed both the magnitude and the correlates of cognitive decline in a series of PD patients without depression or dementia during a 3-year follow-up period. There was a significant decline in scores of verbal memory, executive functions, and general cognition during the 3-year follow-up period, and the magnitude of cognitive decline was significantly associated with a late onset of parkinsonian signs, relatively low motor improvement with l-dopa therapy, and the presence of dystonic dyskinesias.

A similar significant association between age at onset of motor symptoms and prevalence of dementia was reported in several cross-sectional studies. Katzen et al. (1998) studied a series of 222 PD patients using a cognitive assessment that tested visuospatial skills, memory, and executive functions. A regression analysis demonstrated that an older age of disease onset consistently predicted cognitive deficits. Glatt et al. (1996) examined risk factors for dementia in a series of 52 non-demented PD patients and 43 PD-demented patients. A multiple logistic regression analysis demonstrated that lack of education, severity of motor deficit, and PD onset at age greater than 60 years were all significant predictors of dementia in PD, and together had a positive predictive value of 98%. However, cognitive problems may also be found among patients with an early onset of PD. Wermuth et al. (1996) compared a series of PD patients younger than 56 years and a group of normal controls matched for age, social function, and global cognitive function, and found significantly more severe deficits in short memory span, constructional function, and logical visual sequential cognition in PD patients compared with the control group.

The lateralization of parkinsonian signs was reported to be significantly related to specific cognitive deficits in PD. Tomer et al. (1993) demon-strated that patients with a left-side onset of motor symptoms (i.e., right hemisphere pathology) performed significantly worse on tests of verbal memory, verbal fluency, naming, visuospatial analysis, abstract reasoning, attention span, and mental tracking than patients with a right-side onset of motor symptoms. These findings were replicated by some but not all authors (Starkstein et al., 1987; St Clair et al., 1998). Starkstein and Leiguarda (1993) examined the presence of cortical and subcortical atrophy as assessed with CT scan in a series of 9 patients with bilateral PD, 12 patients with left-hemi PD, 12 patients with right-hemi PD, and 12 age-comparable normal controls. Patients with bilateral PD had significantly more severe cortical and subcortical atrophy than the control group, but there was also a significant association between the side with most promi-nent parkinsonism and more severe contralateral brain atrophy in patients with right- (but not left-) hemi PD. There was also a significant correlation between neuropsychologic deficits and atrophy in specific cortical and subcortical areas: atrophy in the region of the basal ganglia was significantly correlated with perseverations on a test of set-shifting (the Wisconsin Card Sorting Test); deficits on a task of visual memory significantly correlated with atrophy in right and left opercular areas, and deficits of verbal fluency significantly correlated with diffuse cortical and left opercular atrophy.

Finally, the role of genetic factors in the mechanism of dementia in PD was recently examined. In a study that included 146 non-demented PD patients, 120 PD-demented patients, and 903 normal subjects, Marder et al. (1999) found that siblings of PD-demented patients were three times as likely to develop AD as siblings of normal subjects. When only siblings aged over 65 years were considered, there was a five-fold increase in risk of dementia. Based on these findings, the authors suggested a familial aggrega-tion of AD and PD with dementia. Dujardin et al. (1999) examined whether normal first-degree relatives of patients with familial PD (defined as the presence of PD in the proband and in at least one first- or second-degree relative) had signs of neuropsychologic dysfunction compared with normal individuals without first-degree relatives with PD. They found a subgroup of relatives of PD patients with deficits on a test of executive functions of a magnitude comparable to the one reported in early PD, and suggested that cognitive impairment without motor dysfunction could characterize the pre-symptomatic stage of PD in familial PD. One limitation of the study is that follow-up evaluations were not carried out, and whether those relatives with executive dysfunction finally developed full-blown PD could not be ascertained.

In conclusion, older age, a later age at onset of motor symptoms, a longer duration of illness, low education, the lateralization of parkinsonism, and atrophy in specific cortical and subcortical brain regions may constitute significant risk factors for dementia in PD.

Specific cognitive deficits in PD

A wide variety of cognitive deficits were described in non-demented PD patients, with relatively more severity in visuospatial and executive functions and relatively less impairments in memory and speech (Levin & Katzen, 1995). However, given the progression of cognitive deficits along the stages of the illness, the question arises as to whether these specific cognitive deficits are isolated findings or whether they may constitute the initial symptoms of a full-blown dementia. To answer this question, Goldman et al. (1998) compared cognitive and motor functioning in non-demented PD patients, patients with PD and questionable dementia, and a group of normal elderly controls. As expected, the PD group with questionable dementia had significantly more severe cognitive deficits than both the non-demented PD group and the normal control group, but the important finding was that the non-demented PD group showed significantly more severe deficits on tests of verbal memory, constructional praxis, naming, sequencing, and visuospatial scanning compared with the normal control group. Based on this finding, Goldman et al. (1998) suggested that PD may be associated with mild but widespread cognitive deficits, and may predispose to further cognitive decline. Similar findings were reported by Mohr et al. (1990b) in a study that included a selected group of PD patients of "exceptional professional standing" who continued to work successfully in their premorbid occupation and who denied any cognitive impairment. The main finding was that this selected group of PD patients had significant deficits on tasks of episodic memory and visuospatial function compared with normal controls. We will now examine the most prevalent types of specific cognitive deficits reported in PD.

Executive functions

Executive functions refer to the mental processes involved in the realization of goal-directed behavior, such as abstract thinking, planning, ability to profit from feedback, judgment, and initiative (Mohr et al., 1995). The tasks most frequently used to assess this cognitive domain are the Wisconsin Card Sorting Test (Nelson, 1976), which measures the ability to develop and apply new concepts and subsequently shift sets, and the Controlled Oral Word Association Test (verbal fluency) (Benton, 1968), which examines access to semantic information under a time constraint. Deficits in executive functions, and especially in both the Wisconsin Card Sorting Test and verbal fluency, were consistently reported in the early stages of PD (Lees & Smith, 1983; Cooper et al., 1991). On the other hand, Mohr et al. (1990b) could not find significant deficits on a range of tasks that assessed executive functions in a series of high-functioning PD patients, even though these patients had deficits on tasks that assessed episodic memory and visuospatial functions. These findings suggest that deficits in executive functions in PD may be part of a more extensive cognitive decline, or alternatively, that there may be a subgroup of PD patients with deficits restricted to executive functions as the initial manifestation of cognitive problems (Graham & Sagar, 1999).

Dubois and Pillon (1997) suggested that executive dysfunction in PD may result from several factors, such as deficits in behavioral control and regulation, inability to elaborate internally guided behavior, and deficits in processing resources and internal control of attention. They suggested an important role for the striatum in executive functions, since these structures seem to participate in the maintenance of mental set and in focusing attention on single events. In a recent study, Owen et al. (1998) assessed cerebral blood flow changes in PD patients and normal controls using a modified Tower of London planning task. They found a similar prefrontal cortical activation in PD patients and normal controls, but whereas the control group also showed activation on the internal globus pallidus, the PD group showed a significant decrease in the same region. The authors suggested that dopamine depletion in PD may disrupt planning functions by modifying the pattern of striatal outflow from the internal pallidum to frontal cortical areas.

In conclusion, deficits on tests of executive functions may be related to basal ganglia dysfunction. Whereas some studies suggest that executive dysfunction occurs early in the disease, other studies suggest that these deficits are present in the context of additional cognitive impairment.

Visuospatial deficits

The true prevalence of visuospatial impairment in PD remains a debated issue, ranging from studies reporting deficits in most non-demented PD patients to those showing flawless performances in early PD (Levin & Katzen, 1995). One explanation for these discrepant findings is that a wide variety of cognitive tasks with eventually different mechanisms, such as those assessing visual discrimination, visual recognition, visual attention, spatial memory, and spatial planning, have all been subsumed under the label of "visuospatial skills" (Levin & Katzen, 1995). Furthermore, most visuospatial tasks that were assessed on PD patients are time-dependent and make high demands on manual dexterity, which may bias results towards a worse performance among patients with more severe motor deficits. In fact, those studies that used visuospatial tasks adapted to the motor limitations of PD found only mild deficits. Canavan et al. (1990) reported that patients with mild PD had significantly more deficits on a prism adaptation task compared with normal controls, Montgomery et al. (1993) found mild visual perceptual problems in a group of PD patients with mild disease, and Cooper et al. (1993) reported visuomotor constructive deficits in the early stages of PD. Levin et al. (1991) assessed 184 PD patients and 90 age- and education-comparable normal controls using a visuospatial assessment that included tests of facial recognition, line orientation, mental object assembly, visual embedded figures, and block design. Significant between-group differences were found only for the facial recognition test, with a worse performance for the PD group. Crucian et al. (1999) reported significant difficulty with visuospatial processing in PD patients compared with age- and education-matched controls. These deficits were not accounted for by elemental perceptual deficits or the severity of motor disorder. The authors suggested that visuospatial deficits in PD may result from executive dysfunction and disruption of frontal basal ganglionic and frontoparietal systems.

Related to the issue of visuospatial deficits in PD is the concern about driving ability in this disorder. Heikkilä et al. (1998) assessed driving ability in 20 PD patients and 20 age- and gender-matched controls using cognitive and psychomotor laboratory assessments and a structured on-road driving test. The main finding was that PD patients had some deficits on the driving ability tasks, although most of them were also found to be sufficiently competent to drive. Both the patients' neurologists and the patients themselves overestimated their driving ability: 35% of the patients who received their neurologist's approval to drive failed to pass the driving test, although they were still driving actively. The major driving problems of PD patients were found in the context of heavy traffic in an unfamiliar city. There was a highly significant correlation between the cognitive laboratory tests and the driving test, and slowness of cognitive processing was considered to be the main cognitive correlate of driving problems. The authors suggested that the evaluation of driving ability in PD patients should include tests of vigilance and concentration, visual perception, choice reaction time, and information processing in a complex situation.

In conclusion, non-demented PD patients may show mild deficits on some visuospatial tasks such as prism adaptation, visual perception, visuomotor construction, and facial recognition. Given that some of these tasks may require active planning and strategy formation, deficits in executive functions may account for some of the early visuospatial impairment in PD. Driving abilities may be impaired even in the early stages of the illness, and should be assessed with appropriate instruments.

Speech and language

The most prevalent speech problems in PD are hypophonia (i.e., reduced variability in pitch and loudness) and dysarthria (i.e., deficits in word articulation), with a decreased use of vocal parameters for achieving stress and emphasis (Illes, 1989; Ackermann & Ziegler, 1996). PD patients may also show tachyphemia (i.e., an acceleration of speech rate), and less commonly, compulsive repetition of words and phrases. Illes (1989) assessed spontaneous language in five patients with PD and reported silent hesitations at the beginning of sentences. He suggested that these deficits may be secondary to impairments in planning upcoming linguistic sequences. Ho et al. (1999) examined the ability of PD patients to regulate speech volume in different contexts. PD patients had deficits in increasing their overall speech volume in accordance with the pragmatics of the conversational task, which were considered to be due to impairments in the appreciation of the pragmatic aspects of speech.

PD patients may also show repetitive speech phenomena, characterized by speech iterations with repetition of syllables, words, or phrases. Benke et al. (2000) reported palilalia (hyperfluent and poorly articulated iterations, uttered with increasing speech rate and decreasing loudness) and a type of stuttering (a non-fluent, well-articulated iteration pronounced with constant loudness and rate) as the most frequent types of repetitive speech phenomena in PD. These speech abnormalities were mostly present in patients with advanced PD, both in On and Off states.

Prosodic aspects of speech consist of the emphasis placed on certain syllables, changes in tempo or timing, and differences in pitch and intonation, which help to convey semantic and affective information (Lloyd, 1999). Whereas the speech production of patients with PD has been classically described as flat, monotonous and dysprosodic (Darkins et al., 1988), deficits in the identification of prosody were also reported. Blonder et al. (1989) found that PD patients in the early stages of the illness had deficits in the recognition of the emotional intonation of phrases compared with age-comparable normal controls. Similar deficits in the identification of affective prosody in PD were reported by some (e.g., Borod et al., 1990; Pell, 1996), but not all, investigators (e.g., Caekebeke et al., 1991). In a recent study, Lloyd (1999) assessed phonological discrimination, lexical access, semantic comprehension, discrimination, and comprehension of lexical stress, as well as discrimination, comprehension, and identification of affective and linguistic prosody in a series of 16 PD patients without cognitive impairment. Lloyd replicated the finding of deficits of prosody identification in PD, but could not find deficits in phonological, lexical, or semantic tasks.

The extent of language deficits in PD is controversial. Cummings et al. (1988) found significant deficits in tasks that assessed information content of spontaneous speech and comprehension of complex commands in a group of non-demented PD patients compared with age-comparable normal controls. On the other hand, no significant between-group differences were found on other linguistic tasks (e.g., naming comprehension, repetition, reading). Levin et al. (1989) found that patients in the early stages of PD performed similarly to age- and education-matched normal controls on tasks of vocabulary and word retrieval, but showed significant deficits on a task of verbal fluency. Cooper et al. (1991) assessed language deficits in a series of 60 non-demented PD patients who never received dopaminergic agonists, and 40 age-comparable normal controls with similar IQ scores to the PD group. They found mild but significant deficits in PD compared with normal controls in tasks of language expression, object word fluency, and category alternation. Lewis et al. (1998) assessed a series of PD patients and age-matched normal controls with a range of language and cognitive tests. They found that PD patients with intact cognition had a normal performance on tasks of verbal fluency, semantic association, use of synonyms and antonyms, and the production of novel sentences from given information. On the other hand, PD patients with cognitive deficits showed significant deficits on language tasks that also require executive functions, such as verbal reasoning skills, divergent language production, cognitive–linguistic flexibility, and linguistic problem-solving abilities. Semantic deficits were reported in PD patients with mild cognitive deficits, but not among those without cognitive impairment (Portin et al., 2000).

In conclusion, whereas patients with PD may show prominent speech problems, such as dysarthria, hypophonia, and start hesitations, language deficits are milder. Among non-demented PD patients, language functions are relatively preserved, except for mild deficits in verbal fluency and complex language tasks. More severe language problems in PD may be related to an incipient global cognitive decline.

Bradyphrenia

"Bradyphrenia" is the term used to refer to the "slowing of the thinking process" or the "lengthening of normal information processing time" that was suggested as paralleling the motor slowness of PD (Brown & Marsden, 1990). Several studies demonstrated a significant cognitive slowing in PD patients (Mayeux et al., 1987; Cooper et al., 1994) and suggested that bradyphrenia may be the cognitive manifestation of dopamine deficiency. However, whereas Pillon et al. (1989) did replicate a significant slowing on a task that assessed cognitive speed in PD, they could not demonstrate significant improvements upon treatment with l-dopa.

Other studies suggested that bradyphrenia in PD may be related to concomitant mood disorders or global cognitive impairment. Rogers et al.

(1987) examined 30 PD patients matched for age and education, 30 depressed patients without PD, and 30 normal controls. PD patients in this study were assessed before starting any dopaminergic treatment. Using tasks of differing cognitive difficulty, they found a longer cognitive processing time in PD patients compared with the control group, but this increment was significant only in those PD patients with depressive symptoms. When PD patients were re-tested after starting dopaminergic treatment, there was a significant correlation between improvement in the cognitive task and improvement in the patients' depression ratings, suggesting an association between bradyphrenia and depression in PD (the association between depression and cognitive impairments in PD is further discussed in chapter 5).

Several studies using tests of memory scanning, visual attention, manual movement tasks (Rafal et al., 1984), and abstract reasoning (Helscher & Pinter, 1993) could not demonstrate cognitive slowing in PD. Duncombe et al. (1994) assessed a series of PD patients without dementia or depression using a mental rotation task, which provides a cognitive analogue to real movement independent of concurrent motor slowing, and found that the performance of PD patients was similar to normal healthy controls. Smith et al. (1998) examined slowing of cognitive processes for verbal, quantitative, and spatial information, memory scanning, and central processing time in a series of non-demented PD patients with relatively mild parkinsonism. They found no significant differences between the PD group and normal controls on any task of cognitive slowing, which is in agreement with prior studies showing no cognitive slowing in PD (e.g., Helscher & Pinter, 1993; Davidson & Knight, 1995). Smith et al. (1998) suggested that the slowing of cognitive processing in PD reported in some studies may be related to the potential inclusion of PD patients with mild dementia or depression.

Event-related potentials as a measure of bradyphrenia

Event-related potentials (ERPs) measure cognitive processing that is independent of motor speed. The P300 component of the auditory ERP is a measure that may reflect information-processing-related activities, and was reported to be significantly delayed in dementia (Polich et al., 1986). Starkstein et al. (1989) studied ERPs, reaction time, and movement time in a series of PD patients with severe motor fluctuations and On and Off phases. They found a significant decrement in both the P300 latency and movement time in the On phase compared with the Off phase, but no significant phase differences were found in reaction time and the amplitude of the P300. Tachibana et al. (1997) assessed P300 and reaction times to simple and complex stimuli in patients with PD and normal controls. They found PD patients to have a significantly longer latency for both the P300 and the complex reaction time task, and interpreted this finding as an expression of cognitive slowing for stimulus classification and attentional processes. Since they found no significant association between P300 latency and l-dopa therapy, they suggested that noradrenergic depletion may underlie the defective processing of attention and cognitive information in PD. Robertson and Empson (1999) measured reaction times and ERPs in PD patients and normal controls during the performance of a cognitive task that had a progressive increase in difficulty. They found that PD patients and normal controls had a similar correlation between reaction time and the latency of the ERP, and the increment in task difficulty. However, between-group differences were significant for the P300 latency (significantly increased in PD compared with controls) but not for the reaction times, suggesting that cognitive slowing in PD may occur at the stage of stimulus evaluation but not for response selection.

In conclusion, whereas initial studies reported a significant cognitive slowing in PD, more recent studies suggest that bradyphrenia may be primarily related to poor control of the motor demands of the task, an underlying depression, or incipient cognitive impairment. Several studies reported a significant delay in ERPs in PD patients, but whether this finding is related to the concept of bradyphrenia or to other cognitive functions remains to be empirically examined.

Attention and memory deficits

Several studies examined deficits in explicit memory in patients with PD. Whereas most studies found normal recognition of presented stimuli for both verbal and visuospatial material, significant deficits were found on more effort- and attention-demanding free-recall tasks (Dubois & Pillon, 1997). Based on these initial findings, Ruberg and Agid (1988) suggested that the ability to encode verbal or visuospatial material is preserved in PD, whereas the mechanism of recall may be impaired. Dubois et al. (1991)

demonstrated these recall deficits to be unrelated to either age at onset of motor symptoms or the use of dopaminergic agonists, since mild memory deficits were already present in the early stages of the illness in PD patients who were not yet using dopaminergic agonists.

Buytenhuijs et al. (1994) demonstrated that PD patients have a relatively decreased processing of learning strategies that rely on internal generation, and a relatively increased processing of learning strategies that rely on external stimuli. In a recent study, Berger et al. (1999) demonstrated that PD patients with relatively more severe bradykinesia were more dependent on externally guided learning strategies compared with PD patients with less severe bradykinesia.

In one of the most comprehensive studies of memory deficits in PD, Ivory et al. (1999) compared 20 non-demented PD patients and 20 controls with a similar level of physical disability using tests of immediate recall, word list learning in intentional and incidental contexts, word completion priming, remote memory, metamemory, and awareness of mnemonic abilities. PD patients showed significant deficits on new learning of verbal material under incidental (but not intentional) learning conditions, as well as deficits in remote memory and metamemory. On the other hand, no significant between-group differences were found on the remaining memory tasks. Based on these findings, the authors suggested that memory deficits in PD may be attributable to impairments of attention allocation, formulation of retrieval strategies, and effortful learning. Since frontal lobe dysfunction may play an important role in these abilities, Ivory et al. (1999) suggested that memory deficits in PD may be at least partially explained by deficits in executive functions. Similar findings were reported by Pillon et al. (1993), who demonstrated a significant correlation between explicit memory scores and performance on tests of executive functions in a group of patients with mild PD. They suggested that memory deficits may be related to frontal lobe dysfunction, with a preserved ability to register, store, and consolidate information but a defective functional use of memory stores.

Implicit memory is defined as the non-conscious remembering expressed through improved performance of specific operations comprising a particular task with experience. One form of implicit memory is priming, in which performance improvements are directly traceable to previous exposure to specific items. Priming is often assessed by the stem-completion test, in which the patient is asked to complete three-letter word stems, and is evidenced by an increased likelihood of completing the word stem with a previously presented word. Another type of implicit memory is assessed through skill learning, in which performance improvements reflect familiarity or practice with a given task, such as maze tracing. Deficits on tasks of implicit memory were reported in PD, but their severity may depend upon the task being assessed. For instance, PD patients were reported to perform significantly worse than normal controls on a test of completion of incomplete figures, but no significant between-group difference was found on a word-stem completion test (Bondi & Kazniak, 1991). Discrepant findings were also reported on tasks of procedural learning. Pascual-Leone et al. (1993) used a serial reaction time task and found that PD patients required significantly more trials than normal subjects to show procedural learning of long stimulus sequences. Using a different motor skill paradigm, Agostino et al. (1996) could not find significant differences between PD patients and normal controls. Based on these discrepant findings, Sommer et al. (1999) suggested that implicit learning may be only partially impaired in PD, and the magnitude of impairment may be related to the specific task used in the research. The same authors demonstrated that PD patients had significant deficits compared with normal controls on a task of procedural learning consisting of competitive stimuli that require alertness, but not in simple learning procedures such as eye-blink conditioning. Sommer et al. (1999) speculated that patients with PD may show deficits in procedural learning whenever they are aware of the requirement of the task, and suggested that this activity may be mediated through the nigrostriatal dopaminergic system. On the other hand, simple learning procedures (which are normal in PD) may be accomplished through extra-nigrostriatal-frontal pathways. Other studies confirmed that deficits in procedural learning, as assessed by the maze learning test, are not widespread in PD but may be restricted to the specific cognitive requirements of the learning context (Haaland et al., 1997), or to the specific component of the acquisition of skills that is assessed (Koening et al., 1999).

An important question is whether procedural learning in PD is related to the severity of cognitive impairment. Heindel et al. (1989) reported procedural learning to be preserved in non-demented PD patients, but abnormal among those with mild dementia. However, Kuzis et al. (1999)

demonstrated that a specific type of procedural learning was preserved even in demented PD patients.

Working memory consists of a set of information processes used to store, integrate, and update information, especially when performing multiple cognitive tasks (Dalrymple-Alford et al., 1994). Several studies demonstrated working memory deficits in PD (Brown & Marsden, 1990), most evident in tests that require the successful coordination of two concurrent tasks. Owen et al. (1997) assessed a series of PD patients, either medicated with dopaminergic agonists or unmedicated, with a set of tests designed to assess spatial, verbal, and visual working memory. They found that non-medicated PD patients with mild parkinsonism had a normal performance on all three tests of working memory. On the other hand, medicated PD patients with mild parkinsonism had significant deficits compared with normal controls on a test of spatial working memory but not on verbal or visual working memory tasks. Finally, medicated PD patients with severe parkinsonism had deficits on all three working memory tasks. The authors suggested that performance of spatial working memory tasks may depend on the integrity of frontal or medial temporal lobe structures, whereas visual working memory may depend on temporal but not frontal lobe structures. They further proposed that the sequence of working memory deficits may be linked to "the spatio-temporal progression of dopamine depletion within the striatum in relation to the terminal distribution of its cortical afferents." Hodgson et al. (1999) found deficits on a test of visuospatial working memory in patients with mild PD compared with normal controls, and suggested that these deficits may be due to dysfunction of a frontal-basal ganglia circuit subserving spatial working memory. Stebbins et al. (1999) demonstrated that deficits on tests of declarative memory in PD are closely related to the working memory demands of the task (i.e., deficits in declarative memory tests may emerge whenever the task has demands in excess of the limited working memory capacity of the patient).

In conclusion, memory deficits in PD may be related to impairments of recall mechanisms, whereas recognition mechanisms seem to be preserved. Recent studies suggest an important role for executive dysfunction in the mechanism of explicit memory deficits in PD. The performance in tasks of implicit memory and procedural learning may be related to the specific task being assessed, whereas the presence of deficits on tests of working memory may be related to the severity of PD.

Mechanisms of dementia and cognitive deficits in PD

During the past decades a number of studies have examined the neuro-pathologic basis of cognitive deficits and dementia in PD, which were explained as secondary to one of the following: (1) coexisting AD pathol-ogy, (2) diffusion of Lewy bodies to medial temporal and neocortical regions, (3) depletion of dopaminergic neurons in the ventral tegmental area, (4) depletion of cholinergic, noradrenergic, or serotonergic neurons, (5) a combination of some of the above, and (6) other (still unknown) mechanisms. We will address each of these alternatives separately, except for diffuse Lewy body disease, which is specifically considered in chapter 3.

Coexisting AD pathology

In one of the first neuropathologic studies of dementia in PD, Boller et al. (1980) found a significantly higher frequency of AD neuropathology in brains of PD patients with severe dementia compared with normal, age-matched control subjects. The mean density of senile plaques was about 10 times higher than in the control group, and all but one of the PD patients with severe dementia had neocortical fibrillary tangles. On the other hand, patients with mild dementia had no obvious clinicopathologic correlations. Paulus and Jellinger (1991) carried out neuronal counts in the substantia nigra, locus coeruleus, and dorsal raphe nucleus, and reported that PD-demented patients had a significantly higher frequency of senile plaques and neurofibrillary tangles, but no significant differences in subcortical cell counts, compared with non-demented PD patients. Ince et al. (1991) examined the prevalence of AD pathology (i.e., neurofibrillary tangles, senile plaques, and granulovacuolar degeneration) in PD. They found a tendency for a higher prevalence of AD pathology in PD patients compared with controls, but there was no significant association within the PD group between the severity of AD pathology and severity of dementia. Xuereb et al. (1990) reported that about 5–20% of PD-demented patients may show the neuropathologic changes of AD, suggesting that AD changes may account for only a fraction of dementia in PD. Jendroska (1997) examined the relationship of AD pathology to dementia in PD in a study that included fifty postmortem brains of 50 PD patients, 23 of whom were demented. They found "early AD pathology" in a subgroup of PD-demented patients, and found no strong association between AD and PD, suggesting that dementia in PD may result from a combination of cortical and subcortical lesions and pathologic changes in biogenic amine systems. On the other hand, Vermersch et al. (1993) reported that PD-demented patients had a significantly higher concentration of an abnormal Tau triplet (a reliable marker of AD neurofibrillary degeneration) in prefrontal, temporal, and entorhinal cortices compared with non-demented PD patients. Finally, de la Monte et al. (1989) carried out a neuropathologic study of PD-demented patients with or without AD pathology. They found evidence to suggest that PD-dementia with AD changes is due to a combination of both AD pathologic changes in cortical areas, the amygdala, and the hippocampus, and PD changes in the basal ganglia and thalamus. On the other hand, PD-dementia was considered to be primarily subcortical, with restricted involvement of anterior frontal and posterior parietal cortices.

Cortical Lewy bodies

The formation of Lewy bodies in the cerebral cortex has been considered to be one of the most important mechanisms underlying dementia in PD. Yoshimura et al. (1988) reported that PD patients with a history of dementia had a significantly higher density of Lewy bodies in the neocortex compared with PD patients without a history of dementia. Based on similar findings, Burkhardt et al. (1988) suggested that there may be a spectrum of Lewy body disorders, ranging from an asymptomatic form at one end of the spectrum to a full-blown dementia at the other end, and classic PD between these extremes. Churchyard and Lees (1997) examined the density of Lewy bodies, Lewy neurites, neurofibrillary tangles, neuritic plaques, astrocytic gliosis, and neuronal counts in the hippocampus and amygdala of 27 PD patients without AD pathologic changes. They found that the severity of cognitive impairment (as measured by the MMSE) was significantly correlated with the density of Lewy neurites in the CA_2 subregion of the hippocampus. On the other hand, they found diffuse Lewy bodies in only a small proportion of PD-demented patients. Churchyard and Lees (1997) suggested that the pathologic process in the CA_2 hippocampal region may disrupt hippocampal function by interfering with inputs to the CA_1 subregion, and further extension of Lewy bodies into cortical areas may contribute to dementia in PD.

Braak et al. (1998) carried out a neuropathologic study on brains of PD-demented patients and found large numbers of Lewy bodies in the entorhinal cortex, and Lewy neurites in the hippocampus, midline nuclei of the thalamus, anterior cingulate gyrus, anterior insula, temporal cortex, amygdala, and all major biogenic amine nuclei. Braak et al. (1998) stressed that PD-demented patients also presented the neuropathologic changes of AD with concomitant disruption of important limbic circuits, and concluded that AD pathology is the most common cause of dementia in PD. However, recent studies using immunostaining of α-synuclein – a very specific marker of Lewy bodies – led to opposite views. Hurtig et al. (2000) demonstrated that Lewy body neuropathologic changes in the neocortex is the most important pathologic correlate of dementia in PD, and found that neuropathologic changes of AD in cases of PD always occurred together with cortical Lewy bodies. Moreover, Haroutunian et al. (2000) found a significant correlation between the density of Lewy bodies and a global measure of dementia in multiple brain regions, regardless of any additional neuropathology. Mattila et al. (2000) found the number of Lewy bodies in the frontal lobes to be the strongest neuropathologic predictor of cognitive impairment in PD, which was independent of the presence of AD pathology.

Depletion of dopaminergic neurons

The mesencephalic ventral tegmental area contains dopaminergic cell bodies that send projections to subcortical limbic structures (e.g., the nucleus accumbens and amygdala) as well as to limbic-related cortical regions (primarily the orbitofrontal cortex and the cingulate gyrus). Depletion of dopaminergic cell bodies in the ventral tegmental area has been consistently reported in PD (Agid et al., 1987). Dubois and Pillon (1997) suggested that degeneration of the mesocortical dopaminergic system may play an important role in the intellectual impairments of PD, since dopamine concentrations in the prefrontal and entorhinal cortex were found to be significantly lower in demented compared with non-demented PD patients. Rinne et al. (1989) reported a significant association between the severity of cognitive deficits and neuronal loss in the medial portion of the substantia nigra, and dementia in PD patients without concomitant AD pathology has been associated with greater neuronal depletion in the ventral tegmental area

(Zweig et al., 1993) and a significant loss of dopaminergic terminals compared with non-demented PD patients (Agid et al., 1990).

Rinne et al. (2000) carried out [^{18}F] fluorodopa PET studies and a comprehensive neuropsychologic evaluation in a series of 28 PD patients and 16 age-comparable normal controls. They found a significantly lower [^{18}F] fluorodopa uptake in the putamen, caudate and frontal cortex in PD patients compared with controls. They also found a significant association between [^{18}F] fluorodopa uptake and cognitive performance, but only with tests that demanded working memory and attention (i.e., tests thought to be sensitive to frontal lobe functions). Furthermore, those correlations were significant for [^{18}F] fluorodopa uptake in the caudate and frontal cortex, but not for uptake in the putamen or temporal lobe, suggesting that dysfunction of the dopamine system is significantly related to the cognitive deficits of PD. Holthoff-Detto et al. (1997) reported a similar association between lower uptake of [^{18}F] fluorodopa and impaired performance on a delayed recall verbal task.

Depletion of other neurotransmitter systems

Most of the cholinergic innervation to the cerebral cortex and the hippocampus originates in the cell bodies of the septal nuclei and the substantia innominata. PD-demented patients were reported to show a significantly greater neuronal loss in the nucleus basalis of Meynert than non-demented PD patients (Candy et al., 1983), and the magnitude of this neuronal drop-out was found to be similar to that in AD (Arendt et al., 1983). Paulus and Jellinger (1991) found a significant association between mild (but not severe) dementia in PD and neuronal loss in the nucleus basalis of Meynert. They suggested that degeneration of the nucleus basalis may produce mild dementia, whereas more severe dementia may result from AD neuropathologic changes.

Asahina et al. (1998) used PET and the radioligand [^{11}C] N-methyl-4-piperidylbenzilate ([^{11}C] NMPB) to assess muscarinic acetylcholine receptors (MARs) in a series of 12 PD patients and 8 normal controls. They found a significantly higher MAR binding in the frontal cortex in PD patients compared with controls, suggesting loss of pre-synaptic cholinergic neurons. They suggested that cognitive dysfunction in PD may result from cholinergic deficits in the frontal cortex.

Abnormalities in serotonergic and noradrenergic transmission were also considered to have an important role in the mechanism of cognitive deficits in PD. Most of the noradrenergic fibers innervating the cortex originate in the cell bodies of the locus coeruleus. Whereas cell loss in this structure has been consistently found among patients with PD (Mitzutan et al., 1991), those with dementia were reported to show a significantly lower noradrenaline metabolic activity than non-demented PD patients (Cash et al., 1987). Ruberg and Agid (1988) reported a significant association between the level of serotonergic metabolites and receptors in the striatum and medial frontal cortex of PD patients and the magnitude of cognitive deficits. Paulus and Jellinger (1991), however, could not find a significantly greater neuronal depletion in the locus coeruleus or dorsal raphe in demented compared with non-demented PD patients.

Bédard et al. (1998) suggested that depletion of catecholamines could at least partially account for the distractibility and frontal-lobe-like syndrome in PD. They examined the efficacy of the selective noradrenergic α_1-agonist, naphtoxazine, in a series of a PD patients who were assessed on measures of cognition and evoked potentials, and found significant improvements in tasks of attention.

Other mechanisms of dementia

In a clinicopathologic study of 100 PD patients, Hughes et al. (1993) could not find a pathologic cause of cognitive decline in 55% of the PD-demented patients. One limitation of that study was that both the amygdala and the hippocampus were not examined, so it could not be established, whether PD-demented patients had Lewy body or neurites in those areas.

Mechanisms of specific cognitive deficits

The question now arising is whether the specific cognitive deficits reported in some non-demented PD patients have similar neuropathologic underpinnings to those in PD-dementia. Alexander et al. (1986) described five parallel circuits that link the frontal lobe and subcortical structures. These circuits have an origin in specific frontal areas, project to striatal structures such as the caudate, putamen, and ventral striatum, connect these striatal nuclei to specific thalamic nuclei, and close with projections back to frontal areas. One important implication of this system is that disruptions at different points within a circuit may produce similar behavioral effects (Cummings, 1993). The dorsolateral prefrontal circuit originates in the convexity of the frontal lobe and projects to the head of the caudate, which connects to the internal globus pallidus and substantia nigra through a direct pathway, and with the external globus pallidus through an indirect pathway. Both pallidal and nigral structures project to the ventral and dorsomedial thalamic nuclei, which project back to the dorsolateral prefrontal cortex. Bédard et al. (1999) suggested that a reduced dopaminergic modulation of the striatum may disrupt the circuits linking the striatum to the dorsolateral frontal cortex, generating deficits on tasks of executive functions. Dopamine depletion in the caudate is greatest in its most rostral portion, and this area is strongly connected to frontal dorsolateral regions that are implicated in higher cognitive processes, such as planning (Owen et al., 1995). Significant correlations were reported between dopamine transporter density in the head of the caudate and putamen and cognitive tasks that assessed "frontal lobe" functions, such as tests of verbal working memory and executive functions (Muller et al., 2000). There is also dopamine depletion within the frontal cortex that is secondary to degeneration of the mesocortical dopamine system, which may further account for the frontal-like deficits in PD.

Mohr et al. (1995) suggested different mechanisms for the specific cognitive deficits in PD, since not all PD patients with mild cognitive deficits were found to progress to overt dementia. He considers PD to be an heterogeneous disorder, and different neuropathologic changes (e.g., AD or Lewy bodies) or a differential extent of these changes (e.g., diffuse vs focal Lewy bodies) could account for this heterogeneity. In a recent study, Graham and Sagar (1999) examined the clinical heterogeneity in PD using motor, cognitive, affective, and demographic data of a large sample of patients. Based on a cluster analysis, they identified five subgroups of patients:

Group 1 – good motor control without cognitive impairment

Group 2 – good motor control and cognitive deficits restricted to executive functions

Group 3 – an older age of disease onset, poor motor control, and mild global cognitive impairment

Group 4 – poor motor control without cognitive impairment

Group 5 – poor motor control with moderate to severe global cognitive deficits.

Based on these five clusters, Graham and Sagar (1999) suggested three different subtypes of PD: the "motor only" subtype, which may be due to pathology restricted to nigrostriatal dopaminergic pathways; the "motor and cognitive" subtype, which may feature both nigrostriatal and mesocorticolimbic dopaminergic pathology together with other subcortical or cortical alterations; and a "rapid progression" subtype, which may result from multifocal (cortico-subcortical) pathology.

Other mechanisms were also proposed to account for the focal cognitive deficits in PD. Hu et al. (1999) carried out a proton magnetic resonance spectroscopy study in 10 non-demented PD patients and 10 age-matched normal controls. They found significant reductions in the temporoparietal cortex ratio of N-acetylaspartate creatine (NAA/Cr) + phosphocreatine in the PD group compared with the normal controls. This reduction was most evident in the temporoparietal cortex contralateral to the side with relatively more severe parkinsonism, and there was also a significant correlation between the reduction in the NAA/Cr in the temporoparietal cortex and a worse performance on tests of language, executive, and visuospatial functions. Since no follow-up data were available, whether this MR spectroscopy abnormality predicts further dementia could not be determined, but these findings are in agreement with reports of reduced metabolic activity in temporoparietal areas in PD-demented patients (Starkstein et al., 1997; Hu et al., 2000).

In conclusion, about one-third of PD-demented patients show the neuropathologic changes of AD in neocortical areas, the amygdala and the hippocampus, together with the neuropathologic changes of PD in the basal ganglia and thalamus. A high proportion of PD-demented patients show Lewy bodies in neocortical areas and subregions of the hippocampus, amygdala, and all major biogenic amine nuclei. Dementia in PD was also reported to be significantly associated with depletion of dopaminergic cell bodies in the ventral tegmental area and medial portion of the substantia nigra, and with depletion of cholinergic cell bodies in the nucleus basalis of Meynert.

General conclusions

Both overt dementia and deficits in specific cognitive domains have been described in PD. Dementia is present in about 20% of PD patients in cross-sectional samples, but longitudinal studies suggest that a higher proportion of PD patients may develop severe cognitive deficits along the progression of the illness. Dementia in PD was found to be significantly related to the duration of illness, low education, and a late age at onset of parkinsonism. The extent of specific cognitive deficits in non-demented PD patients is still a debated issue. PD patients may show mild deficits on some visuospatial tasks and on learning of verbal material under specific conditions. Concomitant deficits on attention allocation, formulation of specific cognitive strategies, and effortful tasks suggest that impairments of executive functions may account for at least some of the cognitive deficits in PD. Bradyphrenia, or the slowing of cognitive process, has been frequently associated with PD, but recent studies suggest that both depression and incipient cognitive decline may mostly account for that disorder. Neuropathologic findings in PD-dementia are varied. Most cases show Lewy bodies in neocortical and limbic regions, and about 20% of cases may show the neuropathologic changes of AD. On the other hand, significant associations between specific cognitive deficits and restricted brain neuropathology are yet to be found.

Depression in Parkinson's disease

In his *Essay on the Shaking Palsy*, James Parkinson (1817) stated that patients may become demoralized by the disease and may eventually refuse treatment. Janet (1924) was the first to recognize an explicit association between depression and PD, and explained the mood disorder as secondary to psychologic trauma.

In this chapter we will examine the phenomenologic aspects of depression in PD and discuss its prevalence, main clinical correlates, longitudinal evolution, and potential mechanisms. We will begin with a clinical case that features most of the usual manifestations and problems arising from depression in PD.

Clinical vignette

O.B. is a 74-year-old engineer who was referred to a neurology clinic because of gait problems and falling episodes. His motor problems had started 1 year before, when he noticed more rigidity in his right upper and lower limbs and a tendency to fall toward the right. On neurological examination he showed hypophonia, slight loss of facial expression, intermittent resting tremor in his right hand, mild cogwheel rigidity restricted to the right side, mild slowing on finger tapping, hand movements, and leg agility, moderately stooped posture, slow shuffling gait, and mild postural instability. The patient reported that several years before the onset of the motor problems he became more apathetic and lost interest in his everyday activities. At the onset of parkinsonian signs he also developed a depressive mood, and reported feeling sad most of the time, with difficulties in falling asleep, loss of interest in activities of daily living, worrying about minor matters, difficulties in concentration, and loss of energy and libido. He was diagnosed as having PD and major depression, and was started on l-dopa (125 mg q.i.d.) and nortriptyline (with an initial dosage of 25 mg/day and reaching a dosage of 75 mg/day 2 weeks later). Two months after starting treatment, O.B. showed marked improvements in both his motor impairments and his mood disorder.

Table 5.1. Phenomenology of autonomic and psychologic symptoms of depression

Autonomic symptoms	Psychologic symptoms
Autonomic anxiety	Worrying
Anxious foreboding	Brooding
Morning depression	Loss of interest
Weight loss	Hopelessness
Delayed sleep	Suicidal plans
Subjective anergia	Social withdrawal
Early morning awakening	Self-depreciation
Loss of libido	Lack of confidence
	Simple ideas of reference
	Guilty ideas of reference
	Pathologic guilt
	Irritability

Phenomenologic aspects of depression in PD

A vexing problem in neuropsychiatry is how to obtain a valid diagnosis of depression in patients with a neurologic illness when symptoms that are central to the diagnosis of mood disorders may be produced by the neurologic disease itself, independently of the depressive disorder. Patients with PD and patients with "primary" (i.e., no known brain injury) depression may show both bradykinesia and motor retardation, a blank facial expression, apathy, a stooped posture, and sleeping problems. Robinson (1998) raised the question of whether this overlap and potential non-specificity of depressive symptoms in neurologic disorders may require radical changes in the assessment methods, and discussed four different strategies to diagnose depression among the neurologically ill: (1) the diagnosis of depression based on psychological symptoms without consideration of vegetative or autonomic manifestations (Table 5.1), based on the assumption that psychological symptoms may be less likely to be influenced by the physical illness; (2) the clinical judgment about whether autonomic symptoms relate either to the physical illness or to depression; (3) the diagnosis of depression based on those symptoms that were demonstrated to be specific to depression in the disease under study; and (4) the diagnosis of depression based on standardized diagnostic criteria, such as in DSM-IV (American Psychiatric

Association, 1994) or ICD-10 (World Health Organization, 1992), provided that the use of these criteria does not elevate the number of false positives (i.e., patients meeting criteria for depression in the absence of a true depressive syndrome).

The question then arising is whether PD may "produce" symptoms of depression in the absence of a depressive mood. Starkstein et al. (1990c) compared the extent of overlap between symptoms of PD and symptoms of depression by measuring the frequency of autonomic and affective symptoms of depression in PD patients without a depressed mood compared with age-matched non-depressed patients with an acute myocardial infarction. Both groups were assessed with a semi-structured psychiatric interview that included the Present State Exam (Wing et al., 1974). The main finding was that non-depressed PD patients were no more likely to have autonomic or affective symptoms of depression than patients with an acute myocardial infarction, demonstrating that PD in the absence of depression, compared with another medical disorder, does not contribute significantly to the presence of depressive symptoms.

Hoogendijk et al. (1998b) examined the overlap of symptoms due to depression or PD in a study that included 100 PD patients assessed with both a standard inclusive method, which scored the presence of a symptom irrespective of its origin, and a diagnostic–etiologic ("exclusive") method, which excluded symptoms that were considered to be due to PD. Using the inclusive method, major depression was diagnosed in 23% of the patients, whereas this frequency decreased to 13% when using the exclusive method. This finding demonstrates that the strategy chosen to diagnose depression may greatly influence the estimate of prevalence, and raises the issue of specificity of depressive symptoms in PD.

Starkstein et al. (1990c) examined the specificity of psychologic and autonomic symptoms of depression in PD in a study that included 33 patients who reported a depressed mood and 33 patients who denied depressive feelings. Both groups were matched for Hoehn and Yahr (1967) stage, duration of illness, age, and education. Autonomic and psychologic symptoms of depression were assessed using the Present State Exam (Wing et al., 1974). The main finding was that both psychologic and autonomic symptoms of depression, except for "early morning awakening" and "anergia and retardation," were significantly more frequent in depressed PD

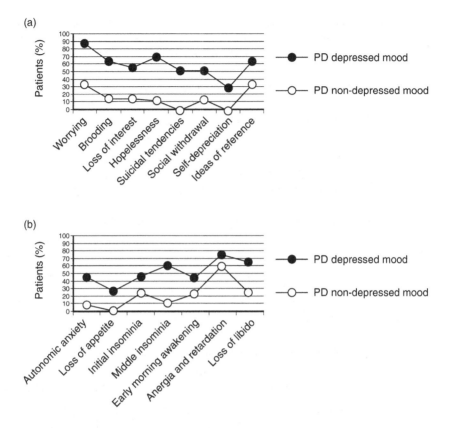

Figure 5.1. Both psychologic (a) and autonomic (b) symptoms of depression, except for "early morning awakening" and "anergia and retardation," were significantly more frequent in depressed PD patients than in non-depressed PD patients.

patients than in non-depressed PD patients (Figure 5.1). A similar lack of specificity of psychomotor retardation was more recently reported by Hoogendijk et al. (1998b). These findings are not surprising since motor retardation, related to bradykinesia and rigidity, is one of the cardinal symptoms of PD. Early morning awakening is also a frequent complaint of patients with PD, and may result from a "wearing-off" phenomenon, morning dystonic movements (which are sometimes painful), or both.

Taken together, these findings suggest that anergia, motor retardation, and early morning awakening should not be included in the criteria used to diagnose depression in PD, and should not be rated on the depression scales used in this population. Based on these findings, Starkstein et al. (1990c)

Table 5.2. DSM-IV criteria for major depressive episode

A. Five (or more) of the following symptoms have been present during the same 2-week
period and represent a change from previous functioning. At least one of the symptoms is
either: (1) depressed mood or (2) loss of interest or pleasure.
  (1) Depressed mood most of the day, nearly every day, as indicated by either subjective
      report or observation made by others.
  (2) Markedly diminished interest or pleasure in all, or almost all, activities most of the day,
      nearly every day.
  (3) Significant weight loss when not dieting or weight gain, or decrease or increase in
      appetite, nearly every day.
  (4) Early insomnia or hypersomnia, nearly every day.
  (5) Psychomotor agitation, nearly every day.
  (6) Feelings of worthlessness or excessive or inappropriate guilt, nearly every day.
  (7) Diminished ability to think or concentrate, or indecisiveness, nearly every day.
  (8) Recurrent thoughts of death, recurrent suicidal ideation without a specific plan, or a
      suicide attempt or specific plan for commiting suicide.

Adapted from DSM-IV.

suggested that the diagnostic criteria shown in Table 5.2 should be used for
the diagnosis of major depression in patients with PD.

The presence of at least three affective and three autonomic symptoms of
depression was reported to have a sensitivity of 96% and a specificity of
100% for the diagnosis of major depression (based on DSM-III diagnostic
criteria) (Starkstein et al., 1990c). Other studies confirmed that both autonomic and psychologic symptoms are common features of depression in
PD (Gotham et al., 1986), and Levin et al. (1988) demonstrated that
autonomic symptoms are specific to the depressive syndrome of PD and do
not constitute a somatic artifact.

The DSM-IV (American Psychiatric Association, 1994) includes the
category of "mood disorder due to a general medical condition" (Table
5.3), which specifies two diagnoses: one with depressive features (if the
predominant mood is depressed but the full criteria for a major depressive
episode are not met), and one with a major depressive-like episode (if the
full criteria for a major depressive episode are met). Thus, when using the
DSM-IV criteria, depression in PD should be diagnosed under this category.

Depression rating scales such as the Hamilton Depression Scale

Table 5.3. DSM-IV criteria for mood disorder due to a general medical condition

A. A prospective and persistent disturbance in mood predominates in the clinical picture and is characterized by either (or both) of the following:
   (1) depressed mood or markedly diminished interest or pleasure in all, or almost all, activities
   (2) elevated, expansive, or irritable mood
B. There is evidence from the history, physical examination, or laboratory findings that the disturbance is the direct physiologic consequence of a general medical condition.
C. The disturbance is not better accounted for by another mental disorder.
D. The disturbance does not occur exclusively during the course of a delirium.
E. The symptoms cause clinically significant distress or impairment in social, occupational, or other important areas of functioning.

Types:
With depressive features: if the predominant mood is depressed but the full criteria are not met for a major depressive episode.
With major depressive-like episode: if the full criteria are met for a major depressive episode.
With manic features: if the symptoms of both mania and depression are present but neither predominates.

Adapted from DSM-IV.

(HAM-D) (Hamilton, 1960), the Beck Depression Inventory (BDI) (Beck et al., 1961), and the Montgomery–Asberg Depression Rating Scale (MADRS) (Montgomery & Asberg, 1979) have been widely used as screening instruments for depressive disorder in PD, and for assessing the relative severity of depressive symptoms. Leentjens et al. (2000) found both the HAM-D and the MADRS to be adequate instruments for measuring depressive symptoms and for diagnosing depressive disorder in PD, but also reported that a single cut-off score on the BDI was not sufficient to separate depressed from non-depressed PD patients with adequate sensitivity and specificity.

In conclusion, both psychologic and autonomic symptoms of depression are specific to the depressive syndrome of PD, except for the symptoms of anergia, motor retardation, and early morning awakening. Ideally, depression in PD should be diagnosed using semi-structured psychiatric interviews, and the severity of depression assessed with valid and reliable depression scales such as the HAM-D and the MADRS.

Prevalence of depression in PD

The prevalence of depression in PD has been reported to range from 7% to 90%, and this wide range may be explained by referral biases in the samples studied. For instance, the highest prevalence of depression (90%) was reported in a study that included patients selected from admissions to psychiatric units (Mindham, 1970), whereas the lowest prevalences of depression were obtained in epidemiologic samples. Hantz et al. (1994) assessed depression in PD patients living in a metropolitan area and found a prevalence of both mood and anxiety disorders of 7%, and a rate of major depression of only 3%. In another community-based study that included 245 patients with PD, Tandberg et al. (1996) found major depression in 8% of the patients, although a further 24% of the sample had depressive symptoms of a moderate severity. Meara et al. (1999) established a community-based register for parkinsonism within a defined geographical area of North Wales. In a random sample of 132 PD patients (excluding those with severe dementia) they found that 64% had severe symptoms of depression, but less than 10% of them were on antidepressant drugs. Finally, in a community-based sample of 97 patients with PD, Schrag et al. (2001) reported moderate to severe depression in 20% of patients.

Studies that examined prevalences of depression in PD patients attending a neurology clinic usually produced higher frequencies of depression compared with epidemiologic samples. In a study that included a consecutive series of 105 patients who were seen in a neurology clinic for regular follow-up visits and were assessed with a structured psychiatric interview, Starkstein et al. (1990b) found that 20% had major depression and 21% had minor depression. Using the same psychiatric assessment, Brown and MacCarthy (1990) examined 40 patients with PD and found a high frequency of simple depression, tension, irritability, worrying, and loss of interest and concentration. Seventy percent of the patients had at least one of these symptoms, whereas 55% had two or more symptoms. In a study that included a consecutive series of 101 Chinese patients, Liu et al. (1997) reported a prevalence of major depression of 18% and "other depressive disorders" (mostly dysthymia) in another 25%. Davous et al. (1995) found major depression in 9% of a series of 506 PD patients attending the neurology services in French general hospitals.

Another methodologic variable that may account for some of the discrepancies in the prevalence of depression in PD is the type of assessment used, since higher prevalences of depression were obtained with semi-structured psychiatric evaluations such as the Present State Exam or the Structured Clinical Interview for DSM-IV (Spitzer et al., 1992), whereas lower prevalences were reported in studies using simpler screening instruments or depression rating scales.

In conclusion, about 40% of PD patients may meet criteria for depression in cross-sectional samples, but prevalences may vary according to case ascertainment (epidemiologic vs hospital-based samples) and sampling methodology (cut-off scores on depression scales vs standardized diagnostic criteria based on semi-structured psychiatric interviews).

The course of depression in PD

Two important questions about depression in PD are, first, whether depression may occur before the onset of motor symptoms, and second, how long depression lasts when left untreated. In a sample of 34 patients with recent-onset PD, Santamaria et al. (1986) found that 10 out 11 patients with a depressive syndrome had the onset of depression before the onset of motor symptoms. In a cross-sectional study of depression in a consecutive series of 105 patients attending a neurology clinic, Starkstein et al. (1990b) found that 29% of those with major depression were depressed before the onset of motor symptoms, compared with only 5% of PD patients with minor depression and 2% of PD patients without depression ($P < 0.001$).

Another interesting finding in Santamaria et al.'s (1986) study was that those PD patients who were depressed at the time of the evaluation were significantly younger at the onset of parkinsonian symptoms than nondepressed PD patients. These findings were later confirmed by Starkstein et al. (1989a), who reported that PD patients with an onset of motor symptoms before the age of 55 years had a significantly higher frequency of major depression than patients with a late onset of symptoms (after age 55). This difference remained significant even after early- and late-onset groups were matched for duration of illness. In the early-onset group, depression scores correlated significantly with the severity of cognitive impairment, whereas within the late-onset group depression scores correlated significantly with impairments in activities of daily living (ADLs).

Several studies examined the prevalence of depression in the different stages of PD. In their cross-sectional study of 105 PD patients, Starkstein et al. (1990b) divided the sample into groups belonging to each of the five Hoehn and Yahr stages of the illness. Prevalences of depression were 40% in stage I, 19% in stage II, 36% in stage III, 65% in stage IV, and 50% in stage V. In stage I, the frequency of depression was significantly associated with the side that manifested symptoms (i.e., patients with parkinsonism on the right side showed a significantly higher frequency of depression than patients with symptoms on the left side), and severity of depression correlated significantly with l-dopa dosage. In late stages of the disease there was a significant correlation between depression scores and deficits in ADLs (i.e., more severe deficits in ADLs were associated with more severe depression), suggesting either that impairment, when it becomes quite severe, leads to depression, or that depression leads to a greater degree of impairment in ADLs.

In a prospective 1-year follow-up study, Starkstein et al. (1992) found that 56% of patients with major depression at the initial evaluation still had major depression at follow-up, 33% had a minor depression, and 11% were not depressed (Figure 5.2). Notably, less than 10% of these depressed patients were on antidepressants at the time of the follow-up evaluation. Among patients with an initial diagnosis of minor depression, 26% still had a minor depression at the 1-year follow-up evaluation, 11% had a major depression, and 63% were not depressed (Figure 5.2). Finally, among patients that were not depressed at the initial evaluation, 82% were not depressed at the 1-year follow-up interview, and the remaining 18% had a minor depression (Figure 5.2). These findings allow the following conclusions: (1) whereas most major depressions in PD were found to last for about 1 year, minor depressions are significantly shorter-lasting; (2) the finding of new depressive episodes in about 20% of the sample in a 1-year period suggests that most patients with PD may show depression at some point during the longitudinal evolution of the illness.

In conclusion, depression may start before the onset of motor symptoms of PD, and mostly occurs among patients with an early onset of PD. Major depression in PD may last for more than 1 year, whereas minor depression

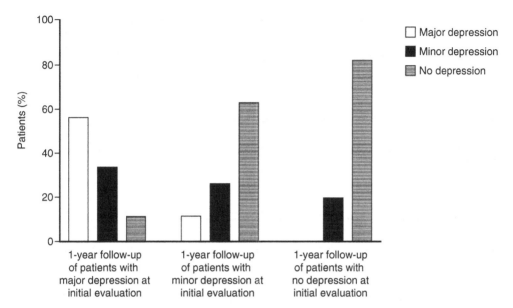

Figure 5.2. Most PD patients with major depression at the initial evaluation were still depressed at follow-up, whereas most PD patients with minor depression at the initial evaluation were not depressed at follow-up.

is shorter-lasting. Most patients with PD may eventually develop depression at some point during their longitudinal evolution. Whereas in the early stages of the illness depression is significantly related to symptom location and l-dopa dosage, in the late stages depression is significantly related to impairments in ADLs.

Physical disability and depression in PD

The high prevalence of depression in PD may be explained as secondary to the severity of physical limitations (i.e., the more severe the impairment the more severe the depression). In this scenario, the prevalence of depression should be greatest in the late stages of the illness, when impairments are most severe. Cole et al. (1996) studied whether depression contributes to impairment in function independently of the severity of parkinsonian signs, and found a weak association between depression scores and illness severity. In men, depression was significantly correlated with physical impairments and social functioning, but these correlations were not significant for

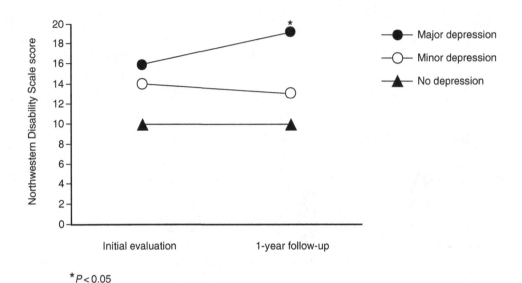

*P < 0.05

Figure 5.3. PD patients with major depression had a significantly greater decline in activities of daily living (represented by an increase in Northwestern Disability Scale score) after a 1-year follow-up compared with patients with either minor or no depression.

women with PD, thus arguing against a simple explanation of depression as secondary to the physical impairments of PD. In a recent study, Schrag et al. (2001) reported that depression was more strongly related to the patients' perceptions of handicap than to actual disability.

To disentangle the association between depression and physical impairments, several studies examined longitudinal changes in mood and ADLs in PD. In their 1-year follow-up study, Starkstein et al. (1992) found that PD patients with major depression had a significantly greater decline in ADLs than PD patients with either minor or no depression (Figure 5.3). Moreover, PD patients with major depression had a significantly faster progression along the stages of the illness than minor or non-depressed PD patients: by the 1-year follow-up, 67% of the major depressed patients had progressed to the next Hoehn and Yahr stage, compared with 41% of the patients with minor depression and 20% of the non-depressed patients ($P < 0.01$).

Brown et al. (1988) examined changes in depression and disability scores across time in a study in which patients were assessed at an average of 14 months apart. At the initial evaluation they found a significant, albeit small, correlation between depression and disability (i.e., the more severe the depression the more severe the disability). Patients who were not depressed at the initial evaluation but became depressed at follow-up were among the least disabled at the initial evaluation, but showed a significantly greater increase in disability at the follow-up evaluation compared with non-depressed PD patients who were still non-depressed. Brown et al. (1988) interpreted this finding as suggesting that PD patients with a slowly progressing disability may show a low prevalence of depression owing to their having enough time to adapt, whereas patients with a faster evolution of disability may be more vulnerable to depression. Alternatively, these findings may be interpreted as showing that the presence of depression produces further physical disability.

The association between depression and specific parkinsonian signs has rarely been studied. Starkstein et al. (1998) examined the association between depression and the cardinal motor symptoms of PD (i.e., tremor, rigidity, and bradykinesia) in a study that compared 78 patients with classic PD (featuring tremor, rigidity, and bradykinesia) and 34 patients with the akinetic–rigid variant (featuring rigidity and bradykinesia, but not tremor). The main finding was that patients with akinetic–rigid PD had a significantly higher prevalence of major depression than patients with the classic variant (38% vs 15%, respectively; $P < 0.01$), but no differences were found in the prevalence of minor depression. Schrag et al. (2001) recently reported a significant correlation between more severe depression and higher akinesia scores. Kuhn et al. (1996a) examined the influence of depression on fine motor skills in 54 PD patients (half with and half without depression). They found the depressed PD group to have a worse performance on quick, complex arm-hand movements compared with non-depressed PD patients, and speculated that the worse performance in depressed PD patients may be the result of either poor motivation or deficits in fronto-subcortical motor loops.

In conclusion, most studies to date showed a significant, albeit mild, correlation between depression and physical disability in PD. Whether disability produces depression, or a depressive state results in more severe disability, has not been clearly established. Follow-up studies suggest that patients with major depression have a significantly faster decline in ADLs and a faster progression along the stages of the illness compared with non-depressed PD patients. Depression is significantly more prevalent in akinetic–rigid PD compared with classic PD and is associated with more deficits in fine motor skills, suggesting an interesting interaction between the mechanism of depression and specific motor signs of PD.

Cognitive impairments and depression in PD

Cognitive impairments are frequently found among patients with PD (see chapter 4) and depression was reported to account for some of these deficits. Starkstein et al. (1990b) reported that PD patients with major depression ($n = 21$) had significantly lower Mini-Mental State Exam (MMSE) scores than non-depressed PD patients ($n = 64$), but no significant differences on MMSE scores were found between minor-depressed and non-depressed PD patients. A regression analysis demonstrated that depression scores accounted for most of the variance with MMSE scores, whereas other factors such as age, duration of illness, severity of impairments in ADLs, and parkinsonian signs accounted for a lesser part of the variance.

Tandberg et al. (1997) assessed a community-based sample of 245 PD patients and found that impaired cognitive function (as defined by a MMSE score of < 24) and thought disorder (as defined by a score of 2 or more on the respective item of the Unified Parkinson's Disease Rating Scale (UPDRS) (Fahn & Elton, 1987)) increased the probability of major depression by a factor of 6.6 and 3.5, respectively. They also found significant correlations between depression scores and more severe impairments in ADLs, presence of motor fluctuations, higher daily dosages of l-dopa, and younger age.

Starkstein et al. (1989c) examined whether depression in PD is significantly associated with a specific profile of cognitive deficits in a study that assessed the Wisconsin Card Sorting Test (which measures the ability to develop new concepts and shift sets), the Controlled Oral Word Association Test (which examines access to information with time constraint), the Trail Making Test (which examines visual, conceptual, and visuomotor tracking), the Symbol Digit Modalities (which examine visual–verbal substitution speed), the Design Fluency Test (a non-verbal counterpart to the Controlled Oral Word Association Test), and the Digit Span (which examines auditory attention) in 15 PD patients with major depression and 15 PD patients without depression matched for age, education, and Hoehn and Yahr stage of illness. The main finding was that PD patients with major depression showed a significantly worse performance in tasks related to executive functions, such as the Wisconsin Card Sorting Test, the Controlled Oral Word Association Test, the Design Fluency Test, and section B of the Trail Making Test compared with PD patients without depression. On the other hand, when a group of 19 patients with minor depression was compared with its respective, matched, non-depressed PD group, no significant between-group differences were found on any of the neuropsychologic tests. Similar findings of no significant differences between minor-depressed and non-depressed PD patients on cognitive tasks were reported by other authors (Boller et al., 1998), suggesting that depression-related deficits in executive functions in PD are specific to major depression.

Cognitive deficits were also reported in patients with primary (i.e., no known brain dysfunction) major depression, raising the question of whether PD patients with major depression may show cognitive deficits beyond those reported in primary major depression. To examine this issue, Kuzis et al. (1997) assessed, with a comprehensive neuropsychologic evaluation, a series of 31 non-depressed PD patients, 19 major-depressed PD patients, 27 patients with primary depression, and 13 age-comparable normal controls. Patients with major depression, with or without PD, showed significantly more severe deficits on tests of verbal fluency and auditory attention than non-depressed patients with PD or age-comparable normal controls. However, PD patients with major depression showed significantly more severe deficits on tasks of concept formation and set-shifting than the other three groups. These findings demonstrate that, whereas some cognitive deficits in major-depressed PD patients may be fully explained by the presence of depression, deficits in concept formation and set-shifting may be related to neuropathologic changes that are specific to PD with major depression.

The question then arising is whether major depression and the progression of the disease may independently account for the cognitive deficits in PD. To examine this dual influence of depression and stage of illness, Starkstein et al. (1989c) assessed with a neuropsychologic test a consecutive series of 94 PD patients who were divided into groups with mild PD (i.e., Hoehn and Yahr stages I and II), moderate PD (i.e., stage III), and severe PD (i.e., stages IV and V). Each group was further subdivided into those with depression (either major or minor), or no depression. A three-factor analysis of variance showed a significant effect for severity of illness: patients in the group with severe PD showed a significantly greater cognitive impairment than the other groups. There was also a significant effect for depression: depressed patients performed significantly worse than non-depressed patients. Finally, there was a significant interaction between severity of illness and presence of depression: depressed patients in the group with severe PD showed significantly greater neuropsychologic impairment than the other groups, and these impairments were most marked in tests that assessed executive functions.

The finding of a significant association between depression, cognitive impairments and severity of illness does not answer the question of whether cognitive deficits may result from more severe depression or vice versa. To examine this issue, Starkstein et al (1990a) assessed 49 PD patients on two occasions 3–4 years apart. Eighteen of them were depressed at the initial evaluation and 31 patients were not depressed. Whereas both groups showed similar MMSE scores at the initial evaluation, the depressed group showed a significant decline over the 3–4 year period compared with the non-depressed group (Figure 5.4). Moreover, the presence of depression was associated with a subsequent loss of intellectual function even when the depression was no longer present. Another interesting finding was that patients treated for depression had only an 11% decrease in cognitive scores compared with a 23% decrement in cognitive scores for non-treated depressed patients, suggesting that adequate treatment of depression may be of potential help in preventing or delaying the progression of cognitive deficits in PD.

In a separate study, Starkstein et al. (1992) examined whether PD patients with either major, minor or no depression had a similar cognitive decline over a 1-year period. Whereas all three groups had a similar MMSE score at the initial evaluation, 1 year later the major-depressed group had a significant decline in MMSE scores compared with both the minor and the non-depressed groups. Taken together, these findings suggest two forms of depression – one with major depression followed by a rapid cognitive

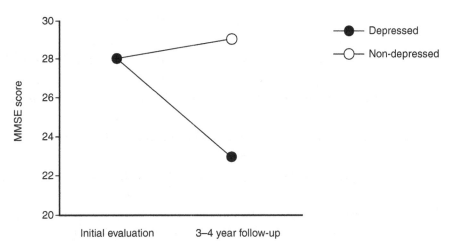

Figure 5.4. Whereas depressed and non-depressed PD patients had similar MMSE scores at the initial evaluation, the depressed group showed a significant decline over a 3–4 year period compared with the non-depressed group.

decline, and one with minor or no depression in which the cognitive decline is more gradual.

In conclusion, depressed patients with PD have significantly more severe cognitive deficits than non-depressed patients, and this association seems to be specific for major depression. Depression-related cognitive deficits in PD were primarily found in executive functions. PD patients with major depression had more severe cognitive deficits than patients with primary major depression, and also demonstrated a significantly faster cognitive decline than minor or non-depressed PD patients.

Other correlates of depression in PD

Sleep problems and pain are frequent complaints among patients with PD, and may be related to night-time motor disability and both akinesia and painful dystonia during sleep induction. Starkstein et al. (1991) examined the association between sleep problems, pain and depression in a study that used separate questionnaires to assess sleep quality and the presence and severity of pain. The main finding was that PD patients with major depression had significantly more sleep problems and pain than PD patients with minor or no depression. Whereas PD patients with minor depression had significantly more severe sleep problems than non-depressed PD patients, no significant between-group differences were found in the severity of pain. A multiple regression analysis, which included scores of sleep problems and pain as the dependent variables and age, duration of illness, severity of parkinsonian signs, l-dopa dosage, and depression scores as independent variables, demonstrated that depression scores accounted for most of the variance with pain and sleep scores, suggesting that at least some of the sleep problems and pain in PD may be epiphenomena of an underlying depression. Sleep problems in PD may also be associated with other psychiatric problems. Pappert et al. (1999) recently reported a significant association between sleep problems and hallucinations in a consecutive series of 126 PD patients, and suggested that improvements in sleep quality in PD may also reduce hallucinatory behaviors.

Several studies reported significant sexual dysfunction in PD (Brown et al., 1990; Lipe et al., 1990). Brown et al. (1990) suggested several potential causes for the high prevalence of sexual problems in PD, such as the prominent autonomic dysfunction in the disease, diminished physical capacity, depression and low self-esteem, and the caregiver's stress and fatigue. They assessed a group of PD patients and their partners with scales of sexual function and associated variables, and found sexual dysfunction in 65% of their male patients and in 52% of their partners. The most common problems were infrequency of sexual intercourse, poor communication with the spouse, and anorgasmia. Male patients also showed a high frequency of erectile problems and difficulties in ejaculatory control. One-third of patients with sexual problems considered the motor symptoms of the disease to be the main cause of their deficits. There were also significant associations between sexual problems and the severity of anxiety and depression, and between the severity of the spouse's sexual problems and the severity of the patient's own strain. On the other hand, there were no significant associations between the patients' sexual problems and the level of physical disability, l-dopa dosage, or autonomic dysfunction.

Whereas Brown et al.'s (1990) study consisted mainly of male patients, Welsh et al. (1997) assessed sexuality in 27 women with PD. Compared with 27 normal controls, women with PD had significantly less satisfaction with their sexual relationship, greater anxiety or inhibition during sex, greater vaginal tightness, and a high frequency of involuntary urination. The authors considered the high prevalence of sexual dysfunction in women with PD to be related to the patients' dissatisfaction with their body appearance, increased preoccupation with their health, and the relevance of medical problems. However, depression was present in 52% of the women with PD compared with 15% of the controls, suggesting that depression may also play an important role in the sexual dysfunction of women with PD.

In a recent study, Kuopio et al. (2000) examined the quality of life in a community-based sample of 228 patients using a specific rating scale. The main finding was that depression was the variable associated most significantly with the experienced quality of life, whereas deteriorating clinical stage, increasing duration of the disease, and lower cognitive capacity had less importance. Similar findings were reported by Schrag et al. (2000), who found that depression, disability, postural instability, and cognitive impairment had the greatest influence on quality of life in their series of PD patients.

In conclusion, sleep problems, sexual dysfunction, and pain are frequent complaints among patients with PD. Depression seems to play an important role in the mechanisms of these symptoms, and is the most important correlate of quality of life in PD.

Biological markers of depression in PD

The dexamethasone suppression test (DST) consists of the administration of 1 mg of dexamethasone orally, which, in normal conditions, suppresses serum cortisol secretion the following day. Caroll et al. (1981) reported that a significant number of patients with melancholic depression fail to suppress serum cortisol secretion after dexamethasone administration. Kostic et al. (1990) examined the usefulness of the DST as a biological marker of depression in PD and found a non-suppressor response in 75% of depressed PD patients and in 28% of non-depressed PD patients. On the other hand, Frochtengarten et al. (1987) reported non-suppression in only 14% of 35 depressed PD patients compared with 5% of the 21 non-depressed PD patients. Mellers et al. (1995) assessed the growth hormone response to apomorphine in PD patients and found that depression was a significant predictor of both average and peak growth hormone increase, implicating dopaminergic mechanisms in the etiology of depression in PD.

Patients with primary (i.e., no known brain injury) depression were reported to show abnormalities in corticotropin-releasing hormone (CRH) neurons of the hypothalamic paraventricular nucleus, which may be related to the abnormal DST responses in this population (Raadsheer et al., 1995). However, Hoogendijk et al. (1998a) could not find significant differences in CRH neuronal activity between PD patients with or without depression and normal controls, suggesting that depression in PD may have a biological mechanism that is different from that of primary depression.

In conclusion, the specificity of the DST for depression in PD was found to range between 83% and 100%, but the sensitivity ranged from only 14% to 69%. Future studies should examine these discrepancies and assess other potential biological markers of depression in PD.

Mechanisms of depression in PD

Psychologic theories explained depression in PD as an understandable consequence of a chronic and devastating illness (see Brown & Jahanshahi (1995) for a review). As a matter of fact, rigidity and akinesia may impair daily activities such as dressing oneself, toilet activities, and eating; deficits of speech articulation and voice pitch may impair communication, and postural disequilibrium may affect locomotion. Taylor and Saint-Cyr (1990) suggested that the high prevalence of depression in PD patients with an early onset of parkinsonian symptoms may be a reaction to the "illness' detrimental effect on their careers, financial security and quality of life during their most productive years." MacCarthy and Brown (1989) reported that depression in PD was significantly related to the magnitude of disabilities rather than the stage or duration of illness. Feelings of self-worth and the pattern of coping were also related to the severity of depression. Singer (1976) reported that patients with PD had lower incomes and were less likely to work, engage in household tasks, or enjoy a close circle of friends than age-comparable normal individuals. Tison et al. (1997) demonstrated that PD patients had a 10-fold greater dependency in basic ADLs compared with age-comparable normal controls, and during a 5-year follow-up period the institutionalization rate of the PD group was about four times that of the control group. The same study also reported a significant association between depression and increased dependency.

Brown and Jahanshahi (1995) argued that psychologic and social factors make an important contribution to depression in PD. They suggested several key factors for a higher vulnerability to depression in PD, such as the availability and quality of social supports, strategies used to cope with stress, the explanatory cognitions and perceptions of control, and attitudes and beliefs about the self. MacCarthy and Brown (1989) found that all these variables, together with the severity of disability, accounted for most of the variance with depression scores in PD. They suggested that the degree of handicap in PD may be related to life circumstances of the individual, their personal and social resources, and age, and proposed that biochemical factors and handicap may be considered as the two major factors that contribute to depression in PD. Serra-Mestres and Ring (1999) supported this mixed model of depression in PD, suggesting that the pathophysiologic changes associated with PD may lead to an increased vulnerability to developing a "reactive" depression. They examined the performance of non-depressed PD patients in a task that assessed vulnerability to the interfering effects of words with a negative emotional tone. They found that PD patients with higher depression scores performed worse in this task than PD patients with lower depression scores, and speculated that PD patients with higher depression scores may have an increased vulnerability to exter- nal negative emotional stimuli, which may ultimately lead to the develop- ment of clinical depression.

Several studies compared the frequency of depression in PD and in other similarly incapacitating disorders, such as rheumatoid arthritis and hemip- legia. Some of them (e.g., Gotham et al., 1986) showed a similar prevalence of depression in PD patients compared with their respective control group, but others showed a significantly higher prevalence of depression in the PD group. Menza and Mark (1993) assessed the severity of depression and anxiety in a series of 104 PD patients and 61 disability-matched individuals with impaired mobility due to osteoarthritis. The main finding was that PD patients had significantly higher depression and anxiety scores than the control group. Cantello et al. (1986) examined 18 PD patients during both the On (i.e., mobile) period and the Off (i.e., end-of-dose deterioration) period. A control group that consisted of patients with active rheumatoid arthritis with a repetitive pattern of mobile and immobile periods was also assessed. The main finding was that, in both mobile and immobile periods, depression was significantly more severe in the PD group compared with the active rheumatoid arthritis group, even though both groups were comparable in overall physical disability. Pilo et al. (1996) assessed the prevalence of depression in 12 patients with PD and 12 patients with multisystem atrophy (MSA) (a disease that causes parkinsonism with poor l-dopa response). Whereas the MSA group showed more severe motor disability, depression scores were similar for both groups. Fetoni et al. (1999) assessed the prevalence of mood disorders in a series of 12 PD patients and 12 MSA patients matched for age and motor disability. Whereas all PD patients were depressed (six with major depression and six with dysthymia), only two patients with MSA showed depression.

Several other findings argue against an interpretation of depression in PD as secondary to the physical impairments. First, the prevalence of depression is similar in both early stages of the illness (when parkinsonian signs are mild) and late stages (when neurologic deficits are most severe). Second, several studies demonstrated that in about one-third of patients with PD depression begins before the onset of motor symptoms (e.g., Starkstein et al., 1990b). Third, whereas the use of dopaminergic agonists is related to significant motor improvements, there is no parallel mood improvement (Mayeux et al., 1984b). Fourth, the presence of major depression predicts a faster decline in ADLs and a faster progression along the stages of the illness compared with non-depressed PD patients (Starkstein et al., 1992).

The question also arises as to whether there is a genetic vulnerability to developing depression in PD. Starkstein et al. (1990b) found that 23% of PD patients with major depression had a positive family history of psychiatric disorders, compared with 33% of PD patients with minor depression and 24% of PD patients without depression, arguing against an important role for genetic factors in the mechanism of depression in PD.

The finding of relatively more severe deficits in executive functions in major-depressed PD patients (Starkstein et al., 1989c) suggests a role for frontal lobe dysfunction in the mechanism of depression, since executive functions were reported to correlate significantly with metabolic activity in the frontal lobes (Owen et al., 1996). Further support for relatively more severe frontal dysfunction in depressed PD patients was provided by Mayberg et al. (1990) in a study that compared major-depressed and non-depressed PD patients and a group of age-comparable normal controls using [18]FDG-PET. Their main finding was that PD patients with major depression had significantly lower metabolic activity in both caudates and inferior frontal cortex compared with PD patients without depression and normal controls. Moreover, there was a significant correlation between the magnitude of metabolic changes in the inferior frontal cortex and Hamilton Depression Scale scores (i.e., the more severe the depression, the lower the inferior frontal metabolic activity). Ring et al. (1994) compared depressed and non-depressed PD patients using the cerebral blood flow PET technique and found that depressed PD patients had significantly lower frontomedial and cingulate metabolic activity than non-depressed PD patients. They also reported that this pattern was similar to cerebral blood flow changes found in patients with primary major depression.

Mayberg et al. (1997) examined brain metabolic changes in depressed PD patients before and after treatment with the selective serotonin reuptake inhibitor, fluoxetine. Mood improvement after fluoxetine treatment was significantly associated with metabolic increments in the dorsal frontal cortex, and this increase was a normalization of an abnormal metabolic pattern (i.e., reduced dorsal fronto-cortical metabolic activity during the depressed state). There was also a significant metabolic decrease in ventral paralimbic areas after successful fluoxetine treatment. On the other hand, fluoxetine non-responders had increased metabolism in ventral paralimbic areas, suggesting that differential metabolic changes in dorsal and ventral frontal areas may play an important role in the antidepressant effect of fluoxetine in PD.

An important role for biogenic amine changes in the mechanism of depression in PD has also been proposed. Cantello et al. (1989) examined the response to methylphenidate in PD patients with or without depression. They found a significantly lower euphoriant effect of methylphenidate in depressed compared with non-depressed PD patients. Since methylphenidate-induced euphoria is related to an increased dopaminergic synaptic activity in limbic areas, Cantello et al. (1989) suggested that degeneration of the mesolimbic dopaminergic system may play an important role in the production of depression in PD. Torack and Morris (1988) reported a marked loss of dopaminergic neurons in the ventral tegmental area of PD patients with dementia and depression. The ventral tegmental area is the main dopaminergic efferent to limbic subcortical structures (e.g., nucleus accumbens, amygdala), and limbic-related cortical regions (e.g., orbito-frontal cortex, cingulate gyrus). Starkstein (1999) speculated that both depression and cognitive deficits in PD may result from a critical level of frontocortical deafferentation from mesencephalic dopaminergic innervation, combined with similar changes in the nigrostriatal dopaminergic system. These pathologic changes may occur in late stages of the disease, and may explain Starkstein et al.'s (1989b) finding of a significant association in late stages of the illness between cognitive impairments and depression.

A similar mechanism may account for the significant association between depression and the akinetic–rigid variant of PD. Paulus and Jellinger (1991) reported that patients with akinetic–rigid PD had significantly more severe neuronal depletion in the lateral and medial substantia nigra and the locus coeruleus than patients with classic PD. They suggested that the akinetic–rigid variant of PD may result from more severe degeneration of the substantia nigra and the locus coeruleus, and speculated that more severe depletion of the ventral tegmental area could disrupt frontal lobe functions and at least partially explain the cognitive impairments of PD. Based on these findings, Starkstein et al. (1998) suggested that depletion of ventral tegmental area dopaminergic neurons may explain their finding of a significant association between major depression and the akinetic–rigid syndrome, as well as the association between major depression and deficits in frontal-lobe-related functions.

Motor fluctuations in PD are related to dopaminergic imbalances, and several studies examined an association between changes in mood in parallel with fluctuations in motor symptoms. Maricle et al. (1995) examined the effect of l-dopa on mood and anxiety in PD patients with motor fluctuations. They used a double-blind design, with l-dopa or placebo infusions and half-hourly ratings of mood and tapping speed. The main finding was that both mood and anxiety improved significantly more after l-dopa compared with placebo infusion, and this response was dose-related (i.e., the higher the l-dopa dose, the greater the mood improvement). Since mood changes and tapping speed were somewhat discordant, and in some patients the mood improvement preceded the motor changes, Maricle et al. (1995) suggested that mood improvement after l-dopa infusion may not be construed as the sole consequence of improved motor function, but may be related to intracerebral mechanisms of depletion and repletion of dopaminergic pathways. Richard et al. (2001) reported on 16 PD patients with motor fluctuations who completed hourly diaries for 7 consecutive days, documenting their mood, anxiety, and motor states using visual analogue scales. There was no consistent temporal relationship between mood and motor states in most of the patients examined.

Several studies on patients with primary depression, using transcranial sonography, demonstrated a significant reduction of echogenicity in the raphe mesencephalic region (Becker et al., 1994, 1995). This region consists of dopaminergic fibers that originate mainly from the ventral tegmental area, serotonergic projections from the dorsal raphe nucleus, and noradrenergic fibers from the locus coeruleus. Becker et al. (1997) assessed, with transcortical sonography, a series of 30 PD patients and 30 age- and gender-comparable normal controls, and found that depressed PD patients had a significantly reduced echogenicity in the raphe mensencephalic region compared with non-depressed PD patients and normal controls. Becker et al. (1997) interpreted their finding as demonstrating an alteration of ascending and descending biogenic amine pathways in the mechanism of depression in PD. A recent study demonstrated decreased pre-synaptic dopamine function in the left caudate of depressed patients with affective flattening and psychomotor retardation (Martinot et al., 2001).

Bejjani et al. (1999) reported the case of a woman with PD who developed transient and acute depression when high-frequency stimulation was delivered to the left substantia nigra. This stimulation site was 2 mm below the subthalamic nucleus, where stimulation improved parkinsonian signs but did not produce mood changes. The authors speculated that the patient's acute depression probably resulted from stimulation of afferent, efferent or passing fibers within the substantia nigra, or from the inhibition of these fibers. More specifically, they suggested that stimulation may have produced dysfunction of those GABA-ergic neurons that innervate the ventral thalamic nucleus, which sends projections to prefrontal and orbitofrontal cortices.

Mayeux et al. (1984a) showed significantly lower levels of the serotonin metabolite, 5-hydroxyindoleacetic acid (5-HIAA), in the cerebrospinal fluid (CSF) of depressed compared with non-depressed PD patients, and

5-HIAA levels were lowest among patients with major depression. Treatment with a serotonergic precursor not only produced a significant mood improvement but also increased CSF levels of 5-HIAA. On the other hand, dysthymic patients with PD showed no greater reduction of 5-HIAA in CSF levels than non-depressed PD patients with PD, supporting the suggestion that major and minor (dysthymic) depressions in PD may have different mechanisms.

Other studies, however, could not confirm a role for biogenic amine abnormalities in the mechanism of depression in PD. Kuhn et al. (1996b) assessed CSF levels of different biogenic amines (noradrenaline, dopamine, and 5-HIAA) in 26 PD patients. To rule out the potential influence of parkinsonian drug therapy on biogenic amine levels, only "de novo" patients (i.e., patients who had never been on antiparkinsonian drugs) were included. The main finding was that there were no significant differences in the CSF levels of depressed and non-depressed PD patients for any of the neurotransmitters and metabolites examined.

In conclusion, neuroimaging evidence suggests an important role for frontal lobe dysfunction in the mechanism of depression in PD. Dorsal frontal areas show reduced metabolic activity during depression, and increase their metabolic activity to normal levels after successful antidepressant treatment. Other studies suggest a role for mesolimbic dopaminergic and serotonergic dysfunction in the mechanism of depression in PD. Eventually, these abnormalities may converge to a single mechanism, since frontal dorsal areas are richly innervated by dopaminergic terminals that originate in the ventral tegmental area. Given the important relationship between dopaminergic and serotonergic systems, degeneration of dopaminergic terminals in the ventral tegmental area may indirectly result in serotonergic dysfunction. Serotonergic fibers originating in the dorsal raphe project heavily toward frontal dorsal areas, and serotonergic abnormalities may further disrupt activity in dorsal frontal regions.

General conclusions

Symptoms of depression are a frequent finding in PD, and several studies have validated the syndrome of major depression in this disorder. The prevalence of depression in PD ranges from a low of 7–9% in epidemiologic studies using screening instruments for depression, to 40% among patients attending a neurology clinic assessed with structured psychiatric interviews. Two types of depression were described – major and minor depression. Major depression may begin before the onset of motor symptoms, is reported to last more than 1 year, is significantly associated with both deficits in executive functions and the akinetic–rigid variant of PD, predicts a faster cognitive and physical decline, and is significantly related to both reduced frontal metabolic activity and reduced CSF 5-HIAA levels. On the other hand, minor (dysthymic) depression in PD was reported to occur after the onset of motor symptoms, has a shorter duration than major depression, is not related to specific cognitive deficits, is not associated with a faster cognitive or physical decline compared with non-depressed PD patients, and is not related to specific CSF biogenic amine changes. These findings suggest that "biological" abnormalities may account for major depression in PD, whereas psychologic factors may produce minor depression in predisposed patients.

6

Anxiety, phobias, apathy, and premorbid personality in Parkinson's disease

The French neurologist Charcot (1875) was the first to describe a specific emotional profile among patients with PD, and considered that both emotions and hereditary factors may play an important role in the mechanism of PD. During the past five decades numerous studies have examined the presence of typical personality types in PD and findings have been quite varied, from reports denying a "typical" personality profile (Glosser et al., 1995) to those describing PD patients as "industrious individuals with high moral standards" (Camp, 1913). PD itself was described as an "illness of the ambitious, moralistic man" and the result of "suppressed hostility" (Dakof & Mendelsohn, 1986). Some studies described specific personality traits such as industriousness, punctuality, inflexibility, and cautiousness as emerging well in advance of the onset of motor symptoms (Poewe et al., 1983), whereas others described a significant personality change only after the onset of parkinsonian signs (Hubble et al., 1993; Menza et al., 1993a). Together with personality changes and a high prevalence of depression (already discussed in chapter 5), symptoms of anxiety, phobias, and apathy have also been recognized as very prevalent emotional and behavioral disorders in PD.

This chapter will review the evidence on specific personality traits, as well as the prevalence, clinical correlates, and potential mechanisms of anxiety disorders and apathy in PD.

Premorbid personality in PD

Early studies of personality traits in PD were framed on a psychoanalytic perspective. (Hubble & Koller, 1995, provide a thoughtful discussion of these works.) For instance, Janet (1924) explained PD as resulting from psychologic losses or trauma, and the motor symptoms were considered to be physical manifestations of an unconscious behavior. Sands (1942) suggested that repression of instinctive impulses and emotions may somehow result in brain injury and the symptoms of PD. Booth (1948) formulated a similar hypothesis, suggesting that the "masked personality" of PD patients and the motor symptoms of the disease may both result from a failure to keep a balance between self-assertion and "moral exactitude." Other authors suggested that PD patients may have deficits in self-assertiveness dating from early childhood, and interpreted the akinesia and freezing phenomena of PD as a manifestation of their inner inhibitions (Mitscherlich, 1960).

The change in psychiatric perspectives during the 1960s and 1970s led to assessments of premorbid personality in PD using structured psychiatric interviews and standardized diagnoses. Initial studies showed either no evidence of a typical premorbid personality or some commonalities in personality type among patients with PD, such as being less talkative and flexible, more generous, even-tempered, cautious, and overcontrolled before the onset of parkinsonism, compared with non-PD individuals (Hubble & Koller, 1995). In a study that compared patients with PD and healthy normal controls, PD patients were described by relatives as more overcontrolled, depressed, introverted, and inflexible premorbidly compared with the control group (Poewe et al., 1983). However, in a later study in which PD patients were compared with patients with essential tremor, Poewe et al. (1990) could not find significant between-group differences in premorbid personality traits or habits.

Eatough et al. (1990) assessed personality traits and life-events history in 30 patients with early-onset PD and in 25 patients with chronic motor disability due to rheumatoid arthritis. They found that PD patients had significantly lower scores than the control group on the personality traits of psychologic mindedness and flexibility, suggesting that PD patients may be considered as cautious, unassuming, deferential to authority, and as having a more rigid personality. They further suggested that the PD patients' "social interactions are of a more conventional and inflexible nature," and that PD patients are "greater social conformists."

Menza et al. (1990) assessed the prevalence of specific personality traits in

20 PD patients and 20 patients with orthopedic and rheumatologic illness. Personality traits assessed were those of (1) "harm avoidance," characterized by a high sensitivity to adverse stimuli, (2) "reward dependence," characterized by a high sensitivity to signals of reward, and (3) "novelty seeking," characterized by a tendency toward excitement in response to novel stimuli. Individuals that are low on this latter trait may show rigid, stoic, slow-tempered, and orderly behaviors, which fits well with early descriptions of the premorbid personality of PD. Menza et al. (1990) found that PD patients scored significantly lower than the orthopedic group on the novelty-seeking personality dimension, both premorbidly and at the time of the evaluation. On the other hand, no significant between-group differences were found on the dimensions of harm avoidance or reward-dependence. Based on animal research findings showing that pulses of dopamine in specific dopaminergic brain sites, such as the nucleus accumbens and ventral tegmental area, are associated with increased pleasure and rewarding behaviors (Crow, 1972), Menza et al. (1990) proposed that the low levels of basal dopamine in PD may produce low "pulses" of dopamine in rewarding brain areas, with a concomitant decrease in novelty-seeking behaviors. In a subsequent study that included 51 PD patients and 31 orthopedic controls, Menza et al. (1993a) replicated their previous finding of lower scores on the "novelty-seeking" personality trait in PD compared with the control group. They found no significant correlation between novelty-seeking and depression scores, suggesting that the presence of depression in PD may not account for this personality trait.

In a study that included a series of 67 Japanese patients with PD, Fujii et al. (2000) reported significantly lower scores in novelty seeking and significantly higher scores in harm avoidance compared with age-comparable healthy controls. Depressed PD patients were also found to have lower scores on novelty seeking and higher scores on harm avoidance compared with non-depressed PD patients, suggesting that depression may influence these personality traits. Menza and Mark (1994) assessed the severity of both depression and personality profiles in a series of 104 PD patients and 61 disability-matched individuals with impaired mobility due to osteoarthritis. PD patients had significantly higher depression scores than the control group, and there was a significant correlation between depression and the personality variable of harm avoidance. However, whether there were significant differences in personality traits between PD patients and the control group was not reported.

Bell et al. (1994) suggested that the "premorbid PD personality" may be clustered into a "shyness" trait, characterized by introverted, shy, timid, subordinate, less outgoing, and nervous behaviors, and a "repressive defensiveness" trait, characterized by responsible, morally rigid, and law-abiding behaviors. In a study that included elderly normal individuals from the community, they found that 17% of the sample scoring in the top quartile for shyness reported family members with PD compared with a prevalence of 2% among those individuals in the bottom quartile. They suggested that the traits of shyness and defensiveness may indicate a relatively high premorbid reactivity among those individuals prone to develop PD.

Hubble et al. (1993) assessed premorbid versus morbid personality profile in a series of 35 PD patients and a group of 35 age- and sex-matched normal controls. Spouses of both PD patients and controls completed the Personality Inventory (Brooks & McKinlay, 1983), based on how they recalled their spouse both at 5 years before the onset of motor symptoms (i.e., remote evaluation) and at the time of the current evaluation. PD patients were recalled as being less "talkative" and "flexible," and more "generous," "even-tempered," and "cautious," before the onset of motor symptoms compared with normal controls. At the time of the current evaluation, PD patients were considered to be more withdrawn and less independent compared with approximately 10 years before the study, and these changes in current personality were significantly correlated with the severity of parkinsonian signs. The authors suggested that PD patients tend to be more quiet and withdrawn even before the onset of motor symptoms.

Other recent studies, however, could not demonstrate a typical personality in PD. Glosser et al. (1995) used the Neuroticism-Extroversion-Openness (NEO) Personality Inventory (NEO-PI) (Costa & McCrae, 1985) to assess personality profiles in patients with PD and two control groups: one that included patients with rheumatoid arthritis and osteoporosis, and another with AD patients. The NEO-PI assesses five dimensions of stable personality traits: neuroticism (i.e., negative emotional adjustment), extroversion (i.e., stimulation-seeking), openness to experience, agreeability (i.e., positive orientation toward others), and conscientiousness (e.g., organization and persistence). When spouses of patients were asked to complete the NEO-PI as the patient was perceived when she/he was in her/his thirties, no major differences were found between patients with PD, AD, or rheumatoid arthritis. When analyses of spouses' ratings were based on the characteristics of patients' personalities at the time of the evaluation, both PD and AD patients scored significantly lower in the NEO-PI dimensions of extroversion and openness than the rheumatoid arthritis group. Patients' own ratings on the NEO-PI were similar to their spouses' ratings, demonstrating good agreement between patients and informants in ratings of personality dimensions. Based on these findings, the authors concluded that there was "no evidence for a specific personality profile for the PD patients either premorbidly or after the onset of motor symptoms." On the other hand, both PD and AD patients showed less extroversion, organization, goal-oriented behaviors, and adequate emotional adjustment after the onset of illness compared with before the onset of motor or cognitive symptoms, suggesting that individuals with a chronic neurologic disorder are more likely to show a common pattern of behavioral changes, which are not specific to PD.

Heberlein et al. (1998) compared personality traits and mood in twin pairs discordant for PD. Using a structured inventory of 138 questions that assessed 10 traits and two dimensions of personality, they assessed six monozygotic and nine dizygotic twin pairs discordant for PD. The main finding was that twins with PD scored lower than normal controls in "inhibitedness," "somatic complaints," and "emotionality," but there were no significant differences in personality dimensions between twins with or without PD. The only significant psychiatric differences between twin pairs were depression (more severe in the PD twin), and social orientation (the twin with PD had been "less often the leader" in the twin pair).

Mechanism of personality changes

Even though the presence of a typical personality in PD has not been consistently demonstrated, several hypotheses for this potential personality change have been proposed. Menza et al. (1995) examined whether the personality trait of novelty seeking, which is characterized by rigidity, loyalty, and orderliness, is "dopamine-dependent." They assessed the [18F] fluorodopa uptake in the caudate and putamen using PET in a small series of nine PD patients. They found a significant correlation between scores of novelty seeking and fluorodopa uptake in the left caudate, suggesting that the decrease in novelty-seeking behaviors demonstrated by some PD patients may be related to dopamine deficits in this brain structure. Whether fluorodopa uptake was also associated with scores of depression was not reported.

The premorbid personality of PD was also explained as secondary to the neuropathologic process of PD, which may begin by producing changes in personality, followed years later by the specific motor changes of PD (Toddes & Lees, 1985). However, whereas motor changes are almost always found after severe dopaminergic neuronal depletion of the substantia nigra, a specific premorbid personality is not universal in PD. Moreover, for this theory to be correct, premorbid personality traits should worsen along the progression of the disease. However, Hubble et al. (1993) reported that personality traits may change from the premorbid state contrary to the expected "PD personality" since the group of PD patients they studied became more flexible and less generous with the progression of illness.

Alternatively, the so-called "typical PD premorbid personality" may be an artifact produced by the presence of depression. In fact, depression is highly prevalent in PD, and Hubble et al. (1993) demonstrated a significant association between descriptions of premorbid introverted personality and the presence of depression at the time of the evaluation. Depression was also reported to pre-date the onset of motor symptoms in a high proportion of PD patients (see chapter 5), suggesting that a low level of novelty-seeking in PD could be an epiphenomenon of a prodromic depression.

In conclusion, whether there is a specific personality profile in PD has been a debated issue. Early studies suggested a premorbid personality profile characterized by lack of flexibility, obsessiveness, and a rigid behavior. Whereas more recent studies suggest that PD patients may show a low profile of novelty-seeking behaviors, other studies could not find differences in personality between PD patients and individuals with other degenerative illnesses. The assessment of premorbid personality is subject to substantial recall bias, which in PD is further complicated by the impaired motor status and the high prevalence of depression and cognitive impairments.

Anxiety in PD

Most studies that examined the prevalence of depression in PD have reported a high prevalence of anxiety symptoms (e.g., Gotham et al., 1986; Starkstein et al., 1993b), leading to specific studies of anxiety in this disorder. Rubin et al. (1986) reported significant episodic anxiety in 16 out of 210 PD patients (8%); in six of them (34%) anxiety coexisted with major depression or dysthymia. Schiffer et al. (1988) examined 16 depressed patients with PD and 20 depressed patients with multiple sclerosis, and found that PD patients had a significantly higher frequency of both generalized anxiety disorder (GAD) (Table 6.1) and panic attacks compared with the control group. Stein et al. (1990) assessed the prevalence of anxiety disorders in a series of 24 patients with PD. Nine of them (38%) received a DSM-III-R diagnosis of current anxiety disorder: two had GAD, five had a panic disorder and two had a social phobia. Seven of the nine PD patients with anxiety disorders had the onset of anxiety symptoms after the onset of parkinsonism. There were no significant differences between PD patients with or without anxiety disorders in cumulative duration of l-dopa exposure, current l-dopa dose, degree of motor disability, and the presence of On–Off fluctuations. The authors stressed that the prevalence of anxiety disorder in their PD group (38%) was higher than that reported in patients with multiple sclerosis, type I diabetes mellitus, or rheumatoid arthritis.

Starkstein et al. (1993b) examined demographic, neurologic, and cognitive correlates of anxiety in a series of 40 PD patients, and found that 52% met DSM-III criteria for GAD. In the overall group of patients, the severity of anxiety (as measured with the Hamilton Anxiety Scale) (Hamilton, 1959) correlated most significantly with depression scores ($R^2 = 0.69$, $P < 0.0001$), leaving no significant correlations for other variables, such as age, MMSE scores (Folstein et al., 1975), and severity of PD. Seventy-six percent of the anxious patients were also depressed, compared with only four of the 19 non-anxious PD patients (21%), thus demonstrating a significant association between depression and anxiety in PD.

Menza et al. (1993b) assessed anxiety in 42 PD patients and 21 patients with chronic debilitating osteoarthritis. They found that 12 out of the 42 PD patients (28%) met DSM-III-R criteria for anxiety disorders (five patients had GAD, five patients had a panic disorder, one patient had a phobic disorder, and one patient had a non-specific anxiety disorder) compared

Table 6.1. Diagnostic criteria for generalized anxiety disorder

A. There must be a period of at least 6 months with prominent tension, worry, and feelings of apprehension about everyday events and problems.

B. At least four of the symptoms listed below must be present, at least one of which must be from items (1) to (4):

Autonomic arousal symptoms

(1) Palpitations or pounding heart, or accelerated heart rate

(2) Sweating

(3) Trembling or shaking

(4) Dry mouth (not due to medication or dehydration)

Symptoms involving chest and abdomen

(5) Difficulty in breathing

(6) Feeling of choking

(7) Chest pain or discomfort

(8) Nausea or abdominal distress

Symptoms involving mental state

(9) Feeling dizzy, unsteady, faint, or light-headed

(10) Feeling that objects are unreal (derealization), or that the self is distant or "not really here" (depersonalization)

(11) Fear of losing control, "going crazy," or passing out

(12) Fear of dying

General symptoms

(13) Hot flashes or cold chills

(14) Numbness or tingling sensations

Symptoms of tension

(15) Muscle tension or aches and pains

(16) Restlessness and inability to relax

(17) Feeling "keyed up," on edge, or mentally tense

(18) A sensation of a lump in the throat, or difficulty in swallowing

Other non-specific symptoms

(19) Exaggerated response to minor surprises or being startled

(20) Difficulty in concentrating, or mind "going blank," because of worrying or anxiety

(21) Persistent irritability

(22) Difficulty in getting to sleep because of worrying

Adapted from DSM-IV.

with one out of the 21 controls ($P < 0.0001$). An additional 40% of the PD group had anxiety symptoms but no formal diagnosis of anxiety disorders. PD patients also showed a significantly higher prevalence of depression compared with the control group (43% vs 14%, $P < 0.05$). Anxiety scores correlated most significantly with depression scores, and neither illness variables (e.g., duration and severity of illness) nor l-dopa dosage explained a significant part of the variance in anxiety scores.

More recently, Aarsland et al. (1999) assessed a variety of neuropsychiatric disturbances in a sample of 139 patients drawn from an epidemiologic study of PD, and found a prevalence of anxiety of 20%. Shiba et al. (2000) examined the association between anxiety and PD in a population-based case-control study that included 196 subjects who developed PD during the years 1976–1995, and 196 healthy control individuals matched by age and gender. They found a higher frequency of anxiety (odds ratio 2.2) and both anxiety and depressive disorders (odds ratio 2.4) in PD cases than in control subjects. Anxiety disorders were significantly associated with subsequent PD even among cases with anxiety occurring 20 or more years before PD onset.

In conclusion, about 30–50% of cross-sectional samples of PD patients may show anxiety disorders (mostly generalized anxiety disorders, and less frequently, panic attacks). Whereas in most patients anxiety occurs comorbidly with depression, some patients may show anxiety symptoms mostly in specific social contexts. This important issue is discussed below.

Anxiety and motor fluctuations

Stein et al. (1990) reported three PD patients who had "social anxiety," which was considered to be secondary to the patients' self-consciousness and embarrassment about their parkinsonian signs. The authors suggested that some of the anxiety symptoms of PD may be related to the motor fluctuations of the disease. Siemmers et al. (1993) assessed anxiety symptoms with the Speilberger Anxiety State and Trait Inventories in a series of 19 PD patients with motor fluctuations. These scales measure the intensity of anxiety at any given moment (state inventory), and the general level of anxiety as a relatively enduring tendency (trait inventory) (Speilberger, 1970). Patients were also examined during On and Off states with a scale that assessed the severity of tremor, walking problems, and difficulty with upper limb movements. The main finding was a significant increment of state anxiety scores during the Off period. This was most evident among patients with clear On–Off fluctuations, suggesting that at least part of the anxiety shown by PD patients may be related to the motor fluctuations of the disease (i.e., more anxiety with less mobility). Maricle et al. (1995) assessed changes in anxiety symptoms in eight PD patients with motor fluctuations during the infusion of two dosages of l-dopa (either a high or a low dosage) or placebo. After the high-dose l-dopa infusion there was a prompt decrement in anxiety scores, whereas the low-dose infusion produced a slower anxiety reduction.

Mechanism of anxiety

The high prevalence of anxiety in PD may be explained as a psychologic response to the physical burden of a chronic and progressive illness. However, Schiffer et al. (1988) found a significantly higher frequency of anxiety in PD patients compared with patients with multiple sclerosis and comparable physical impairment, and neither Starkstein et al. (1993b) nor Menza et al. (1993b) could demonstrate a significant association between anxiety and severity of illness.

Charney et al. (1998) described a "fear and anxiety-producing" circuit, which consists of an afferent arm relaying sensory information through the thalamus, the processing of sensory data in specific cortical (orbitofrontal) and subcortical sites, and the production of behavioral responses through an efferent arm which activates autonomic, neuroendocrine, neurochemical, and neuromotor effectors. They suggested that dysfunction of dopaminergic and noradrenergic pathways may be implicated in the production of anxiety. Since dopamine decreases the firing rate of the locus coeruleus (Cederbaum & Aghajanian, 1977), Iruela et al. (1992) speculated that the loss of dopamine inhibition of the locus coeruleus may underlie the presence of anxiety in PD. Labarca et al. (2001) reported on genetically transformed mice with a severe deficit of dopaminergic neurons upon aging and hypersensitive receptors to choline. These mice displayed increased anxiety, poor motor learning and excessive ambulation that was reduced by low levels of nicotine, suggesting that an abnormal cholinergic–dopaminergic interaction could play a role in the mechanism of anxiety in PD.

A third possibility is that anxiety may be a feature of most depressions in

PD. Whereas several studies identified small groups of PD patients with anxiety disorders but no depression, most anxious PD patients were consistently reported to have a comorbid depression (Menza et al., 1993b; Starkstein et al., 1993b).

In a recent study, Menza et al. (1999) examined depression and anxiety in PD as a function of the variation in the polymorphism in the promoter region of the serotonin transporter gene, which has been linked to anxiety in non-PD individuals. The serotonin transporter was found to be abundantly expressed in the cortical and limbic areas of the brain that are involved in emotional aspects of behavior (Hensler et al., 1994). Menza et al. (1999) found that PD patients with a deficient allele for the serotonin transporter had significantly higher depression and anxiety scores than patients with the more efficient allele, and suggested that the short allele of the serotonin transporter gene may be a risk factor for anxiety and depression in PD.

In conclusion, most anxiety disorders in PD are associated with an underlying depressive mood, suggesting that both anxiety and depression in PD may have a common mechanism. Other studies showed a significant association between anxiety and motor state (i.e., higher anxiety in the Off state), as well as more anxiety in social situations where the patient may feel embarrassed about his or her motor deficits, suggesting that in some PD patients anxiety may be an emotional response to the motor handicap in the context of specific social situations.

Panic disorder in PD

Clinical vignette

N.L., a 54-year-old woman and owner of a small business, was brought in for neuropsychiatric consultation by a friend, who said that N.L. had been very depressed for the previous 6 months. N.L.'s depression had started 3 years previously, when her mother had become very ill. Six months after the onset of depression, she developed writing problems, sudden episodes of breathing difficulties, palpitations, tremor, chills, chest discomfort, dizziness, and fear of dying. These episodes lasted for about 15 minutes, and occurred about twice a week. She slowly developed postural instability, and worried about falling while showering. She started to avoid washing her hair and taking showers, stopped driving, and avoided crowded places. At the interview she reported feeling depressed, with loss of interest in her business, difficulties with concentration, and social withdrawal. Upon physical examination she had a moderate right-side resting tremor, moderate cogwheel rigidity on her right limbs, and moderate bradykinesia on her right hand. She was started on nortriptyline 25 mg/day (which was slowly increased up to 75 mg/day), clonazepam 0.25 mg b.i.d, and l-dopa + benserazide 125 mg q.i.d. One month later the patient reported to be much improved, with normal mood and no anxiety or panic attacks. She started to drive again and began to work with her previous skill and energy. There was also a significant motor improvement, with very mild tremor but no rigidity or bradykinesia. This mood and physical improvement was still evident 1 year after the initial evaluation, without further changes in her medication during this time-period.

A panic attack is defined as a discrete period of intense fear or discomfort, in which a variety of symptoms develop abruptly and reach a peak within 10 minutes (Table 6.2). The most frequent symptoms are palpitations, sweating, trembling, sensations of shortness of breath, choking, chest pain, nausea, dizziness, derealization, fear of losing control, fear of dying, paresthesias, and chills. Vazquez et al. (1993) assessed the prevalence of panic attacks in a series of 131 PD patients, and found that 31 patients (24%) had panic attacks – 9 with "minor" episodes (i.e., few symptoms) and 22 with "major" episodes. Patients with panic attacks had an earlier age at onset of PD, more severe gait disorder, and higher depression and anxiety scores than PD patients without panic attacks. Most panic attacks started about 2 years after the onset of motor fluctuations; the average number of panic attacks was 2.6 episodes per day, and the episodes were strongly related to l-dopa intake and the presence of motor fluctuations (90% of the panic attacks occurred during the Off state). Vazquez et al. (1993) suggested that panic attacks in PD may be related to an abrupt decrement of dopaminergic action upon striatal receptors, with the consequent release of the locus coeruleus from a tonic inhibitory control, and a central surge in noradrenergic transmission.

Fleminger (1991) assessed 13 patients with parkinsonian signs on left limbs only (left hemisphere pathology, LHP) and 17 patients with parkinsonian signs on right limbs only (right hemisphere pathology, RHP); both groups were matched for age, duration of symptoms, disability, severity of parkinsonism, and l-dopa dosage. He found that the LHP group had significantly more severe anxiety and depression than the RHP group. Five of the LHP patients also had panic attacks compared with none in the RHP group.

Yohimbine is a drug that activates noradrenergic neurons by blocking α_2-adrenergic autoreceptors, and was consistently reported to produce panic attacks in patients with panic disorder but not in normal controls (Charney et al., 1984). In a recent study Hegeman-Richard et al. (1999)

Table 6.2. Diagnostic criteria for panic disorder (episodic paroxysmal anxiety)

A. The individual experiences recurrent panic attacks that are not consistently associated with a specific situation or object and that often occur spontaneously. The panic attacks are not associated with marked exertion or with exposure to dangerous or life-threatening situations.

B. A panic attack is characterized by all of the following:
   - it is a discrete episode of intense fear or discomfort;
   - it starts abruptly;
   - it reaches a maximum within a few minutes and lasts for at least some minutes;
   - at least four of the symptoms listed below must be present, one of which must be from items (a) to (d):

Autonomic arousal symptoms
(a) Palpitations or pounding heart, or accelerated heart rate
(b) Sweating
(c) Trembling or shaking
(d) Dry mouth (not due to medication or dehydration)

Symptoms involving chest and abdomen
(e) Difficulty in breathing
(f) Feeling of choking
(g) Chest pain or discomfort
(h) Nausea or abdominal distress

Symptoms involving mental state
(i) Feeling dizzy, unsteady, faint, or light-headed
(j) Feeling that objects are unreal (derealization), or that the self is distant or "not really here" (depersonalization)
(k) Fear of losing control, "going crazy," or passing out
(l) Fear of dying

General symptoms
(m) Hot flashes or cold chills
(n) Numbness or tingling sensations

Adapted from DSM-IV.

carried out a yohimbine challenge in six PD patients with anxiety, and found that three out of five patients with a history of both anxiety and major depression developed a panic attack. They concluded that PD patients with anxiety may respond to yohimbine in a similar way to patients with anxiety disorders but no PD, suggesting a similar underlying mechanism for anxiety disorders in both conditions. However, the study involved only a small sample of patients, and future confirmatory studies may not be feasible given that most patients had a significant rise in blood pressure after yohimbine challenge.

In conclusion, "true" panic attacks may not be a frequent finding in PD, although some panic-like symptoms may occur in about 10% of patients. These symptoms may be an autonomic response of predisposed groups of anxious PD patients when exposed to situations in which their motor problems result in important functional handicaps.

Apathy in PD

Apathy was defined as the absence or lack of feeling, emotion, interest, concern, or motivation (Marin, 1991), and was reported to be a frequent behavioral change among patients with dementia (Starkstein et al., 1995), PD (Starkstein et al., 1992), or strokes to specific brain regions (Starkstein et al., 1993a). One of the major limitations to the study of apathy in neurologic disorders is the lack of adequate structured interviews or standardized diagnostic criteria, but several rating scales have been recently developed (see Appendix). Starkstein et al. (1992) assessed 50 patients with PD using the Apathy Scale, and based on a cut-off score on this scale they diagnosed apathy in 42% of the sample. They also found that two-thirds of the apathetic patients were also depressed. Upon cognitive testing, PD patients with apathy showed significantly more severe deficits on tasks that assessed executive functions and verbal memory compared with non-apathetic PD patients. On the other hand, there were no differences between PD patients with or without apathy in demographic variables, duration of illness, and severity of symptoms of PD, suggesting that apathy may not be simply related to progression of the disease.

In conclusion, apathy appears to be a frequent behavioral change in PD, either alone or comorbidly with depression. Future studies of apathy in PD may use valid and reliable criteria, such as those developed by Marin (1991) and modified by Starkstein (2000) (Table 6.3).

Table 6.3. Diagnostic criteria for apathy

A. Lack of motivation relative to the patient's previous level of functioning or the standards of his or her age and culture as indicated either by subjective account or observation by others.
B. Presence, while with lack of motivation, of at least one symptom belonging to each of the following three domains:

Diminished goal-directed behavior
(1) Lack of effort
(2) Dependency on others to structure activity

Diminished goal-directed cognition
(3) Lack of interest in learning new things, or in new experiences
(4) Lack of concern about one's personal problems

Diminished concomitants of goal-directed behavior
(5) Unchanging effect
(6) Lack of emotional responsivity to positive or negative events

C. The symptoms cause clinically significant distress or impairment in social, occupational, or other important areas of functioning.
D. The symptoms are not due to diminished level of consciousness or the direct physiologic effects of a substance (e.g., a drug of abuse or a medication).

Adapted from Marin (1991).

General conclusions

This chapter reviewed evidence for and against a specific premorbid personality in PD. Whereas initial studies based on the psychoanalytic theory described PD patients as "industrious individuals," with "rigid behaviors" and "high moral standards," other studies could not find differences in premorbid personality traits between PD and other chronic degenerative conditions. On the other hand, both anxiety disorders and apathy have been recognized as frequent behavioral problems in PD. In both cases there is a high association with comorbid depression. Panic-like episodes were also reported to be frequent among PD patients with motor fluctuations. However, whether these episodes are true panic attacks or an emotional response of predisposed individuals to the motor fluctuations of the disease remains to be examined.

7

Neuropsychologic and psychiatric side-effects of antiparkinsonian medication

Introduction

Ball (1882) was the first to suggest that psychiatric disturbances could be part of the clinical picture of PD. However, it was not until the advent of dopaminergic medication that a variety of cognitive and psychiatric problems became consistently recognized, and a wide spectrum of behavioral disorders, including euphoria, hypersexuality, delusions, confusion, vivid dreams, hallucinations, and paranoid psychoses, were related to dopaminergic treatment in PD (Goetz et al., 1982).

This chapter will review the main cognitive and behavioral problems usually associated with the use of antiparkinsonian medication in PD, and present a case that illustrates most of the problems to be examined.

Clinical vignette

N.M. was a 54-year-old man with an 8-year history of PD. At the time of the evaluation he was in Hoehn and Yahr stage IV and on 1 g l-dopa, 3 mg pergolide, and intermittent subcutaneous injections of apomorphine due to severe motor fluctuations. This drug combination produced an acceptable amount of On time during the day but with severe dyskinesias. The patient was started on amantadine with the aim of reducing dyskinesias. Several days later, N.M.'s wife found the patient standing naked in front of the window in the middle of the night. He was shouting at an imaginary group of young people who, according to him, were making unpleasant noises. N.M.'s wife turned on the lights and was able to convince him about the unreality of his perceptions. This event is an example of *visual and auditory hallucinations with preserved insight*, also known as "hallucinosis." The dose of amantadine was reduced by 50%, but the patient continued to show abnormal beliefs such as claiming that his wife was having an affair with another man, which is known as *"delusional jealousy."* A week later, N.M. was found at the local airport waving a gun and looking for his wife and an imaginary lover; his speech was garbled and incoherent. This is considered a *"psychotic state."* He was brought to the hospital and both amantadine and pergolide were discontinued. A CT scan, lumbar puncture, and routine blood tests ruled out concurrent medical illnesses, and the patient remained in the On state and awake during the whole night. He was confused and disoriented, but not agitated. During the following day he alternated short sleeping periods with agitated behaviors. He had "vivid dreams," and woke up scared by a group of imaginary doctors that he believed were conspiring with his wife to kill him. This behavior is known as a *"mood-congruent hallucination."* The patient was started on 12.5 mg clozapine per day, and his behavioral disorder gradually improved. N.M. was discharged 5 days later on 1g l-dopa plus 25 mg clozapine at night-time, free of delusions or hallucinations.

Psychosis in PD

The concept of psychosis in PD primarily includes paranoid delusions and hallucinosis, although other types of delusions (e.g., jealousy, "phantom boarder" – see next section) and "true" hallucinations may also be present. The main phenomenologic aspects of psychosis in PD are described below.

Phenomenology of psychosis
Delusions

Delusions are erroneous beliefs that usually involve a misinterpretation of perceptions or experiences. Among the most frequent types of delusions in PD are paranoid delusions (e.g., abnormal persecutory beliefs that embrace individuals and events, such as threats of harm or theft) and, less frequently, the "Othello syndrome" (the belief that the individual's spouse is unfaithful) and the "phantom boarder syndrome" (the belief that unwelcome guests reside in the patient's home). Delusions are considered to be mood-congruent whenever their content is consistent with the typical themes of a depressed or manic mood (e.g., delusions of personal inadequacy, guilt, disease, death, nihilism, or deserved punishment in the context of a depressed mood) and mood-incongruent whenever their content is not consistent with the typical themes of a depressed or manic mood (e.g., persecutory delusions without self-derogatory or grandiose content, or delusions of being controlled in the absence of an affective disorder).

Illusions

Illusions are misperceptions or misinterpretations of real external stimuli, such as hearing the rustling of leaves as the sound of voices, or the feeling of the presence of unidentified people.

Table 7.1. Diagnostic criteria for delirium due to a medical condition

A. Disturbance of consciousness (i.e., reduced clarity of awareness of the environment) with reduced ability to focus, sustain, or shift attention.

B. A change in cognition (such as memory deficit, disorientation, or language disturbance) or the development of a perceptual disturbance that is not better accounted for by a pre-existing, established, or evolving dementia.

C. The disturbance develops over a short period of time (usually hours to days) and tends to fluctuate during the course of the day.

D. There is evidence from the history, physical examination, or laboratory findings that the disturbance is caused by the direct physiologic consequences of a general medical condition.

Adapted from DSM-IV.

Delirium

Delirium is defined as an etiologically non-specific, organic cerebral syndrome that is characterized by concurrent disturbances of consciousness and attention, perception, thinking, memory, psychomotor behavior, emotion, and the sleep–wake cycle. Delirious episodes have an acute onset and a relatively brief duration, and are characterized by impaired awareness of self and surroundings, impairment of directed thinking, disorder of attention with hypo- or hyperalertness, impairment of memory, diminished perceptual discrimination, disturbance of psychomotor behavior with hypo- or hyperactivity, disordered sleep–wake cycle with drowsiness during the day and insomnia at night, and fluctuations in alertness and in severity of cognitive impairment. The DSM-IV criteria for delirium are presented in Table 7.1.

Hallucinations

Hallucinations are sensory perceptions in the absence of identifiable external stimuli. Hallucinations should be distinguished from illusions, in which a real external stimulus is misperceived or misinterpreted. The person may or may not have insight into the unreality of the perception. An individual with auditory hallucinations may recognize that he or she is having a false sensory experience (also known as "auditory hallucinosis"), whereas another person may be convinced of the reality of the sensory experience (i.e., true hallucinations).

Visual hallucinations in PD usually occur as images on a background of clear sensorium, and are most likely to appear when the patient is drowsy or when the lights are dim (Fenelon et al., 2000). PD patients tend to get used to these phenomena and recognize hallucinations as unpleasant but not frightening experiences (Tanner et al., 1983). Visual hallucinations include well-known individuals, family members, and household pets (Moskowitz et al., 1978). Most frequent are visions of shadowy strangers sitting on a sofa or at a dining table, and small children or strangers in the yard (Sanchez-Ramos et al., 1996). Passage hallucinations are frequent in PD, and are characterized by very brief images localized in the periphery of the visual field, which are usually identified as a person or an animal (Fenelon et al., 2000). On the other hand, elementary visual hallucinations such as flickering light, luminous scotomata, and scintillations are rarely present (Sanchez-Ramos et al., 1996).

Vivid dreams

Vivid dreams are frequent in PD and often precede hallucinations, illusions, and delusions (Moskovitz et al., 1978; Nausieda et al., 1982). Twenty-five percent of PD patients were reported to have REM sleep behavior disorder (RBD), which is characterized by loss of normal skeletal muscle atonia during REM sleep, prominent motor activity, and dreams (Olson et al., 2000). RBD was reported to be significantly more frequent in PD patients with hallucinations compared with PD patients without hallucinations (Arnulf et al., 2000). Pappert et al. (1999) reported that 82% of PD patients with hallucinations have a sleep disorder, characterized by low sleep efficiency and reduced total and relative REM sleep time.

Prevalence and clinical correlates of psychosis

Assessment of psychosis and other behavioral disturbances in PD is usually carried out with rating instruments that are frequently used in patients with "primary" (i.e., no known brain injury) psychiatric disorders (e.g., the Brief Psychiatric Rating Scale (Overall & Gorham, 1988)). Friedberg et al. (1998) designed the Parkinsonian Psychosis Rating Scale to assess the severity and changes of psychosis after treatment. This is a short 6-item scale which was shown to be both valid and reliable (Appendix 5).

Visual hallucinations are the most frequent type of hallucinations in PD (Fenelon et al., 2000). Auditory hallucinations are less frequent, and occur primarily in patients with concomitant visual hallucinations and cognitive impairment (Inzelberg et al., 1998). Moskowitz et al. (1978) reported hallucinations in 30% of 88 patients with PD. Sixty-two percent of those patients with hallucinations had only visual hallucinations, 10% had only auditory hallucinations, and 28% had both types of hallucinations.

Graham et al. (1997) assessed the prevalence of psychotic phenomena in a series of 129 PD patients, and found hallucinations and illusions in 25% of the patients. These phenomena were mostly visual, but with an auditory component in 40% of the cases. They found a peak prevalence of hallucinations within the first 5 years after the onset of PD, superimposed on an increasing prevalence of psychosis with duration of illness. Inzelberg et al. (1998) assessed the prevalence of hallucinations in a series of 121 PD patients, and reported hallucinations at the time of the evaluation or within the preceding 2 years in 37% of the sample. Naimark et al. (1996) found that 19% of a series of 101 PD patients had both delusions and hallucinations, 10% had only hallucinations, and 7% had only delusions. They also found that patients' age, duration of PD, presence of dementia, and MMSE scores were significantly associated with the severity of psychosis. Aarsland et al. (1999) assessed the prevalence and correlates of psychosis in 235 PD patients living in a community. The prevalence of hallucinosis was 10%, whereas another 6% of the sample had hallucinations and delusions. Psychotic symptoms were significantly related to age, stage and diagnostic subgroup of PD, severity of depression, and cognitive impairment. In a series of 216 consecutive PD patients, Fenelon et al. (2000) reported hallucinations or hallucinosis in 40% of the patients within the 3 months prior to the evaluation, with a calculated total lifetime prevalence of hallucinations of 46%. PD patients with hallucinosis had significantly higher depression scores compared with PD patients without psychosis, whereas 70% of the PD patients with dementia had visual hallucinations.

Prodromal indicators of hallucinosis in PD were reported to include: concern with bodily function, anxiety, self-doubt and self-depreciation, social alienation, bizarre feelings, and general dissatisfaction (Glantz et al., 1986). Sanchez-Ramos et al. (1996) found that longer disease duration, higher frequency of depression and dementia, and a history of sleep disturbance were significantly related to the occurrence of hallucinations in a series of 214 PD patients. Giladi et al. (2000) confirmed that depression, especially in patients with an early onset of parkinsonian signs, is an important predisposing factor for psychosis.

In conclusion, psychotic phenomena (e.g., hallucinosis, hallucinations, and delusions) were reported in 10–40% of cross-sectional samples of PD patients, but may occur at some point in the disease process in about half of PD patients. Hallucinations are primarily visual, but auditory hallucinations may be present in 10–20% of the patients. Clinical correlates of psychosis in PD are older age, cognitive impairments, depression, early PD, and sleep disorders.

Mechanism of psychosis

Psychosis in PD is usually considered to be secondary to dopaminergic therapy, since most dopaminergic agents used in PD (especially dopamine receptor agonists) have been reported to produce psychosis, which may improve upon dose reduction (Fenelon et al., 2000).

Drug-induced psychoses have been related to functional alterations in dopaminergic projections from the ventral tegmental area (VTA) to the ventral striatum, amygdala, prefrontal cortex, and medial temporal lobes (Cummings, 1992), whereas visual hallucinations during the Off period may result from a withdrawal syndrome, with differential stimulation of cortical dopamine receptor subtypes (Fernandez et al., 1992).

Graham et al. (1997) suggested that the mechanism of psychosis early in PD may be related to relatively more severe denervation supersensitivity in the mesocortical/mesolimbic dopaminergic system, whereas late psychosis in PD may be related to cortical Lewy body pathology, concomitant Alzheimer's disease, or cerebrovascular lesions. They also suggested a role for a relatively overactive serotonergic system in the mechanism of psychosis in PD. Chronic dopamine replacement lowers 5-HT concentrations that lead to post-synaptic receptor supersensitivity, whose stimulation may produce hallucinations. The abnormal dopamine–serotonin interaction in the limbic striatum could also produce psychosis through abnormal glutamate-modulated activity of dopamine neurons in the VTA (Svensson et al., 1995).

On the other hand, dopaminergic agents may be neither necessary nor sufficient to produce psychosis in PD. Visual hallucinations have been reported in 12% of "de novo" PD patients (i.e., those who never received l-dopa therapy) (Teychenne et al., 1986), and not all patients on l-dopa go on to develop psychosis. Based on their finding of a low frequency of psychosis in PD patients with mild-to-moderate motor impairment even when treated with l-dopa, Growdon et al. (1998) speculated that psychosis in PD may result from neurochemical dysfunction beyond the nigrostriatal dopaminergic system. Moreover, there is no dose–effect relationship between dopaminergic treatment in PD and psychosis, and Goetz & Stebbins (1993) found no significant association between hallucinations and plasma levels of dopamine in a series of 11 PD patients. Non-dopaminergic drugs (e.g., anticholinergics) may also elicit psychosis in PD, and other potential causes of hallucinations in PD are neocortical involvement with Lewy body pathology (Perry & Perry, 1995), and cortical cholinergic deficits (Dubois et al., 1990).

Diederich et al. (1998) examined the relationship between poor visual discrimination and visual hallucinations in PD patients with normal visual acuity and no major ophthalmologic disease. They found that PD patients with visual hallucinations had significantly more severe deficits on tests of color perception and contrast sensitivity compared with PD patients without hallucinations. These deficits may alter the visual sensory input and reduce meaningful information. Diederich et al. (1998) further speculated that this partial sensory deafferentation may facilitate hallucinations on account of the release of stored images that are normally suppressed owing to sufficient visual input information. Fenelon et al. (2000) suggested that passage hallucinations may result from a misinterpretation of a brief perception due to disinhibition of an early part of visual processing. Depressed mood may decrease attentional resources and the ability to inhibit irrelevant recognition, and may explain the significant association between depression and hallucinosis in PD. Fenelon et al. (2000) suggested that cognitive deficits may also play an important role in the mechanism of psychosis in PD, since impaired judgment may lead to misinterpretation of sensory stimuli and may impair insight about the reality of the perceptions and beliefs.Given the high frequency of REM sleep behavior disorder in PD patients with hallucinations, Arnulf et al. (2000) suggested that hallucinations in PD may be related to the partial activation of REM mechanisms, whereas delusions in PD may be related to the repeated emergence of dreams during wakefulness followed by the altered perception of reality.

Genetic factors may also play a role in the mechanism of psychosis in PD (Goetz et al., 2001). Makoff et al. (2000) reported abnormalities in the dopamine D_2 receptor gene that may predispose to drug-induced hallucinations late in the course of PD. De la Fuente-Fernandez et al. (1999) examined whether the apolipoprotein E allele is a risk factor for hallucinations in non-demented PD patients. They found that, after adjusting for age, severity of parkinsonism, duration of treatment, dose of l-dopa, and treatment with dopaminergic agonists, there was still a significant association between the presence of the E4 allele and visual hallucinations.

In conclusion, the mechanism of psychosis in PD may be related to dysfunction of dopaminergic mesocorticolimbic pathways, or to an abnormal dopaminergic–serotonergic interaction. Concomitant anticholinergic treatment and cognitive deficits are important risk factors for psychosis in PD, whereas disease duration, sleep fragmentation, REM disturbances, genetic factors and poor visual discrimination may play an additional role.

Neuropsychologic and psychiatric effects of specific antiparkinsonian medications in PD

L-dopa

Moskowitz et al. (1978) demonstrated that dosages of l-dopa sufficient to improve motor function in patients with mild-to-moderate PD have a negligible influence on cognitive functions, and there is no consistent evidence that l-dopa impairs global cognitive abilities in PD patients (Taylor et al., 1986; Pillon et al., 1989; Cooper et al., 1993). On the other hand, enhanced dopaminergic neurotransmission in the striatofrontal pathway could potentially improve some aspects of cognition that involve frontal lobe functions (Shaw et al., 1980; Banerjee et al., 1989; Vaamonde et al., 1991; Miyoshi et al., 1996). For instance, some aspects of impaired planning performance, multiple-choice reaction time, and delayed verbal memory have been reported to improve with increasing doses of l-dopa (Mohr et al., 1987; Pullman et al., 1988). L-dopa withdrawal was reported to impair frontal-lobe-related cognitive functions such as spatial working memory, spatial forward planning, and visual attention (Lange et al., 1992). Kulisevsky et al. (2000) carried out a 2-year open-label study of l-dopa versus pergolide in a series of de novo PD patients with repeated neuropsychologic evaluations. They found both drugs to produce similar improvements on tasks that assessed learning and long-term verbal and visual memory, visuospatial abilities, and executive functions. This cognitive improvement was maintained for about 1 year after treatment onset, but declined 1 year later, suggesting that improvement in cognitive deficits in PD is restricted to some cognitive domains and not sustained in time.

Motor-state-dependent effects on cognition have also been reported (Girotti et al., 1986; Kulisevsky et al., 1996). For instance, patients who learn in either the On or Off states were reported to show a better recall if retested during the same state (Brown et al., 1984; Huber et al., 1987), but other studies could not demonstrate changes in cognition between On and Off states (e.g., Meco et al., 1991).

L-dopa treatment is rarely associated with episodes of mood elevation, ranging from increased well-being to manic and life-threatening behaviors (O'Brien et al., 1971). Premorbid history of mania is a risk factor for disinhibited behaviors following l-dopa treatment (Klawans, 1982; Factor et al., 1995). Hypomania and hypersexuality may occur during On phases, and feelings of well-being may lead to abuse and dependency of dopaminergic drugs (Nausieda, 1985). Increased libido and inappropriate hypersexuality are present in about 1–10% of PD patients on l-dopa (Cummings, 1992), but paraphiliac behaviors are rarely reported (Quinn et al., 1983).

Giovannoni et al. (2000) described the syndrome of "hedonistic homeo-static dysregulation" in PD patients on dopamine replacement therapy. This syndrome is characterized by the progressive intake of increasing quantities of dopaminergic agonists despite increasingly severe drug-in-duced dyskinesias. Patients with this disorder show a hypomanic behavior with psychomotor agitation, euphoria, irritability, hyposexuality, over-spending, food craving, drug hoarding, and social isolation (Table 7.2). Patients at higher risk are men with an early onset of parkinsonian signs and premorbid psychiatric or personality disorder. The behavioral disorder may improve rapidly after reduction of dopaminergic agents, but patients may be left with depression and negative behaviors. The authors suggested the avoidance of intermittent subcutaneous apomorphine, and treating the behavioral disorder with low-to-moderate doses of olanzapine (2.5–10 mg/day).

Pathologic gambling is a failure to resist the impulse to gamble despite severe personal, family, or vocational consequences, and Molina et al. (2000) described 12 PD patients who developed this disorder among a series of 250 consecutive PD patients. These abnormal gambling behaviors occur-red almost exclusively during On periods, suggesting that this behavioral problem may be associated with an increase in dopaminergic tone.

On the other hand, l-dopa was reported not to influence the prevalence of depression in PD (Cummings, 1992). Two-thirds of patients with

Table 7.2. Diagnostic criteria for "hedonistic homeostatic dysregulation syndrome" due to dopamine replacement therapy misuse

A. Parkinson's disease with documented l-dopa responsiveness.

B. Need for increasing doses of dopamine replacement therapy (DRT) in excess of those normally required to relieve parkinsonian symptoms and signs.

C. Pattern of pathologic use: expressed need for increased DRT in the presence of excessive and significant dyskinesias despite being On, drug-hoarding or drug-seeking behavior, unwillingness to reduce DRT, and absence of painful dystonias.

D. Impairment in social or occupational functioning: fights, violent behavior, loss of friends, absence from work, loss of job, legal difficulties, arguments or difficulties with family.

E. Development of hypomanic, manic, or cyclothymic affective syndrome in relation to DRT.

F. Development of a withdrawal state characterized by dysphoria, depression, irritability, and anxiety at reducing the level of DRT.

G. Duration of disturbance of at least 6 months.

Adapted from Giovannoni et al. (2000).

On–Off phenomena were reported to show increased anxiety during the Off state (Nissenbaum et al., 1990), whereas crying, moaning, shouting and screaming, agitation, and panic states were all reported to be very frequent during the Off state (see chapter 6). L-dopa treatment was also reported to be associated with decreased REM sleep, sleep fragmentation with multiple awakenings, and insomnia (Jenkins & Groh, 1970). Goetz et al. (1989) reported a higher frequency of non-nocturnal hallucinations in patients on a controlled release preparation of l-dopa compared with patients on the standard formulation of l-dopa + carbidopa.

Dopaminergic agonists

Psychiatric side-effects were reported to be frequent with ergot alkaloids such as bromocriptine. This compound belongs to the same pharmacologic family as lysergic acid and diethylamide, both powerful serotonergic agonists with strong hallucinogenic properties, which may explain the psychiatric side-effects of most dopaminergic agonists. Jankovic (1985) reported hallucinations in 28% of a consecutive series of PD patients after 28 months of concomitant pergolide mesylate and l-dopa therapy. In a multicenter drug trial of subcutaneous injections of lisuride maleate and concomitant l-dopa therapy, psychiatric side-effects (e.g., hallucinations, psychosis, nightmares, vivid dreams, paranoia) occurred in 47% of patients

(Vaamonde et al., 1991). Oral lisuride maleate, bromocriptine mesylate, and pergolide mesylate have a similar frequency of psychiatric side-effects, although lisuride is associated with relatively more severe sedation (Lieberman et al., 1985).

Apomorphine

Apomorphine hydrochloride may pose a lower risk of psychiatric side-effects than other dopaminergic agonists. Therefore, patients who develop psychiatric side-effects but cannot be withdrawn from dopaminergic agents should be treated with apomorphine infusions. A manic episode was described in a PD patient treated with apomorphine (Przedsorski et al., 1992) and the administration of this compound to monkeys was reported to produce enhanced sexual behavior (Pomerantz, 1992; Absil et al., 1994). In humans, apomorphine has been reported to increase visual erotic stimuli, and penile erection occurs within a few minutes after apomorphine injection (Heaton, 2000).

Amantadine hydrochloride

Timberlake and Vance (1978) reported insomnia, disorientation, nervousness, and confusion in 15% of a series of 351 PD patients treated with amantadine hydrochloride (200 mg/day) and l-dopa. At higher doses of amantadine (up to 300 mg/day), confusion and hallucinations became more frequent, primarily among patients over 65 years of age, and the highest frequency of psychosis was observed after 3–9 months of treatment. Factor et al. (1998) reported three patients on long-term treatment with amantadine who experienced acute delirium after amantadine withdrawal. This confusional state did not respond to clozapine and only improved after reinstitution of amantadine.

Selegiline hydrochloride

The DATATOP study (The Parkinson Study Group, 1990) found a significant delay in the onset of some cognitive deficits, such as a set-shifting and verbal learning in patients treated with selegiline compared with patients treated with placebo. A later report, however, showed no significant effect of deprenyl on cognitive performance (Kieburtz et al., 1994).

Anticholinergic drugs

In a study that included 75 hospitalized PD-demented patients, De Smet et al. (1982) reported a significantly higher prevalence of confusion among patients on anticholinergic drugs compared with those not receiving such drugs (96% vs 46%, respectively). PD patients on anticholinergics were reported to show a poorer performance on tests that measured cognitive shifting and memory compared with PD patients without anticholinergics (van Spaencdonck et al., 1993). In a neuropathologic study of PD, Ruberg et al. (1982) reported a significant reduction in cortical cholinergic terminals secondary to depletion of cholinergic neurons in the substantia innominata, and speculated that the high prevalence of confusion following treatment with anticholinergic agents in PD may be the result of further functional disruption of the cortical cholinergic system produced by these compounds.

In conclusion, whereas psychosis is the most serious side-effect of l-dopa, some patients may show less frequent behavioral changes, such as euphoria, hypersexuality, the syndrome of "hedonistic homeostatic dysregulation," and sleep disorders. The frequency of psychiatric side-effects with dopamine receptor agonists is about two- to three-fold greater than with l-dopa, and these compounds should be used with great care in PD patients with increased risk of developing psychosis. Both l-dopa and dopaminergic agonists have a negligible influence on cognitive functions, but anticholinergic drugs may produce memory deficits and confusional states.

General conclusions

Delusions, hallucinations, illusions, and vivid dreams are frequent findings in PD patients on dopaminergic treatment. Cross-sectional studies show a frequency of 10–40% for psychosis (i.e., delusions and/or hallucinations), whereas the lifetime prevalence of psychosis in PD is about 50%. Delusions are mostly paranoid, whereas hallucinations are primarily visual. Psychosis in PD is significantly related to older age, longer duration of PD, presence of depression and cognitive impairment, and sleep disorders. In addition, psychosis in PD is relatively more frequent in PD patients on dopaminergic agonists, and the mechanism of psychosis in PD may be related to dysfunction of the dopaminergic limbic system, the overactivity of serotonergic pathways, poor visual discrimination, and the presence of REM sleep behavior disorder. Dopaminergic agents may have a small influence upon cognitive functions in PD, but anticholinergic drugs may produce impairments in anterograde memory, and confusional states.

Treatment of psychiatric disorders in Parkinson's disease

In the preceeding chapters we revised the prevalence of psychiatric disorders and behavioral problems in PD. The consensus is that most patients with PD will become depressed at some point in their evolution, that both apathy and anxiety are frequent comorbid conditions of depression in PD, and that PD patients in the late stages of the illness may show a high frequency of delusions and hallucinations. Despite this high frequency of psychiatric disorders in PD, few studies have examined the usefulness of psychoactive drugs in a systematic way, and there is even less knowledge about the efficacy of other treatment modalities, such as psychotherapy or electroconvulsive therapy in these conditions. In this chapter we will examine the most useful treatment modalities for the different psychiatric disorders of PD, giving priority to controlled studies but discussing findings in open-label studies and case reports as well.

Treatment of depression in PD

Despite the high prevalence of depression in PD, which was reported to be about 40% in cross-sectional samples, most PD patients do not receive adequate antidepressant treatment. A survey of The Parkinson Study Group (Hegeman-Richard et al., 1997) revealed that only 26% of PD patients with depression included in their assessment received antidepressant treatment. In a 1- to 2-year follow-up study, Starkstein et al. (1992) found that only about 20% of the depressed PD patients received antidepressant treatment at some point during the follow-up period. Meara et al. (1996) found a 64% prevalence of marked depression in a series of 132 patients with PD, but less than 10% were on antidepressant drugs.

In a meta-analysis study of antidepressants in PD, Klaasen et al. (1995) carried out an extensive search for relevant papers published between 1966 and 1993. They found that only 12 studies had adequate population size, randomization procedures, selection of outcome measures, low level of dropouts, adequate blinding, and appropriate data presentation. A related finding was that most drug studies in PD were designed to measure the effect of antidepressant medication on parkinsonian signs and not on symptoms of depression. Klaasen et al. (1995) suggested that antidepressant treatment in PD patients should follow the same guidelines as the treatment of depression in elderly depressed patients without PD, and that choice of antidepressant medication should be based primarily on a favorable profile of side-effects.

Antidepressant drugs
Tricyclic antidepressants

The tricyclic antidepressants act through their ability to block the reuptake of the neurotransmitters 5-HT (serotonin) and noradrenaline into their respective nerve terminals. Tricyclic compounds are well absorbed following oral administration and most of them have a half-life of approximately 24 hours, which allows for a once-a-day dosing. Nortriptyline is among the most frequently used tricyclic drugs to treat depression in PD (Andersen et al., 1980). This drug may be started with a dose of 10–25 mg/day and gradually increased over 3–4 days until a dose of 75–100 mg/day is reached. Advantages of nortriptyline are a lower association with orthostatic hypotension compared with other tricyclics, and a defined therapeutic range of serum concentration. Other tricyclic agents, such as amitriptyline (Indaco & Carrieri, 1988), desipramine (Laitinen, 1969), and imipramine (Strang, 1965), were also found to produce significant mood improvements in depressed PD patients, although most of these studies do not meet adequate standards. The most common side-effects of tricyclic drugs in PD patients are dry mouth, constipation, and orthostatic hypotension. Less frequent side-effects are sedation, increased intraocular pressure in patients with narrow-angle glaucoma, urinary retention, delirium, and visual blurring. Tricyclics are contraindicated in patients with heart blocks, severe arrythmias, or a recent myocardial infarction. Tricyclic drugs may have dangerous interactions with drugs that may interfere with their hepatic metabolism, such as cardiac depressant drugs, compounds that may precipitate hypertensive crisis, such as monoamine-oxidase inhibitors, and drugs whose mechanism of action may be altered by tricyclics, such as guanethidine, clonidine, and anticoagulants. Thus, before starting treatment with tricyclic drugs, it is important to review the patient's medical history, a recent electrocardiogram, and current medications.

Monoamine-oxidase inhibitors

There are two types of monoamine-oxidase inhibitors (MAOIs): type A inhibitors, which block the catabolism of serotonin and noradrenaline, and type B inhibitors, which block the catabolism of dopamine. Non-selective MAOIs such as phenelzine were reported to be useful in some cases of PD (Hargrave & Ashford, 1992), but their use is not recommended since they may cause a hypertensive crisis when given together with l-dopa. Side-effects of non-selective MAOIs are more frequent and severe than for other antidepressants, and include dizziness, headache, constipation, dry mouth, insomnia, blurred vision, nausea, peripheral edema, and myoclonic jerks. Selective (i.e., type B) MAOIs such as selegiline have been used with some success in depressed PD patients. Doses of selegiline usually range from 10 mg/day to 20 mg/day; at dosages above 20 mg/day selegiline loses its selectivity and inhibits both type A and type B monoamine-oxidase.

A double-blind, randomized, placebo-controlled trial of 10 mg/day selegiline in PD showed a significant decline in Hamilton Depression Scale scores after 3 months of treatment (Allain et al., 1993). One limitation of the study was that patients were not selected based on their meeting criteria for depression. There are some concerns about using selegiline combined with tricyclic antidepressants or selective serotonergic reuptake inhibitors (SSRIs) because of reports of neurologic toxicity (Richard et al., 1997). Selegiline was also reported to cause psychotic symptoms in some PD patients, most often when given together with other dopaminergic agonists (Tom & Cummings, 1998).

Jansen Steur and Ballering (1999) examined the efficacy of the reversible type A blocker, moclobemide, alone or in combination with selegiline in an open-label, 6-week study that included 10 PD patients with major depression. All 10 patients were on a strict tyramine restriction diet and received moclobemide 300 mg daily. There was a significant decrease in depression scores, which was most evident among patients that were on both moclobemide and selegiline. However, only 2 out of the 10 patients showed a greater than 50% decrease in depression scores from baseline, suggesting that moclobemide may be no more effective than placebo in treating depression in PD.

Selective serotonergic reuptake inhibitors

Selective serotonergic reuptake inhibitors (SSRIs) block the reuptake of serotonin, therefore allowing this neurotransmitter to act for an extended time at synaptic binding sites. The usefulness of these compounds in depressed PD patients was not formally assessed in controlled studies, although their lack of anticholinergic side-effects suggests an important role for these drugs. Whereas SSRIs are usually better tolerated than tricyclic drugs, they may produce agitation, anxiety, sleep disturbance, tremor, sexual dysfunction, and headache. Autonomic adverse effects, such as dry mouth, sweating, weight change, or diarrhea, may also occur, and the association with MAOIs is contraindicated. The "serotonin syndrome" has been described in patients taking SSRIs alone or in combination with MAOIs, and is characterized by confusion, myoclonic jerks, tremor, diaphoresis, diarrhea, and incoordination (Sternbach, 1991; Garcia-Monco et al., 1995).

Several case reports could find only a modest antidepressant effect for fluoxetine in PD, together with prominent side-effects such as tremor, akathisia, dystonia, and bradykinesia (Bouchard et al., 1989; Jansen Steur, 1993; Coulter & Pillans, 1995; Tom & Cummings, 1998). These side-effects could result from a serotonergic inhibition of dopamine release from nigrostriatal pathways, and were reported in PD patients exposed to either fluoxetine, paroxetine, or fluvoxamine (Jimenez-Jimenez et al., 1994; Leo, 1996; Hauser & Zesiewicz, 1997). Other studies, however, could not find a worsening of parkinsonian signs upon treatment with SSRIs (Caley & Friedman, 1992; Montastruc et al., 1994; Waters, 1994).

The efficacy of sertraline was assessed in a group of 15 PD patients who participated in an open-label pilot study (Hauser & Zesiewicz, 1997). Sertraline was started at 25 mg/day, and there was a significant decrease in mean depression scores after 7 weeks of treatment. Two of the 15 patients discontinued sertraline owing to side-effects (light-headedness and insomnia, respectively), but there were no significant changes in mean UPDRS scores.

The efficacy of paroxetine on depressive and motor symptoms was assessed in an open-label study that included 33 depressed PD patients (19 with dysthymia and 14 with major depression) (Ceravolo et al., 2000). Paroxetine was started at 5 mg/day and increased gradually up to 20 mg/day, and the treatment was maintained during a 6-month period. Main results of the study were a significant reduction of depressive symptoms and no worsening of parkinsonian signs. Only one patient showed motor problems (marked worsening of tremor), which improved upon discontinuation of paroxetine. Tesei et al. (2000) examined the tolerability of paroxetine in 65 depressed PD patients. Patients were given a starting dose of 10 mg/day, which was increased to 20 mg/day after 4 weeks of treatment. There was a significant mood improvement as measured with the HAM-D, but 13 patients discontinued treatment due to side-effects (increased anxiety in four, nausea in four, increased Off time duration and exacerbation of tremor in two, and agitation, confusion, and headaches in one patient each).

Other antidepressants

Tolcapone is a catechol O-methyltransferase inhibitor that plays an important role in the metabolic inactivation of dopamine and noradrenaline. When tolcapone is coadministered with l-dopa + benserazide, there is a significant increment in the bioavailability of brain l-dopa, and several studies have demonstrated the usefulness of tolcapone in treating the motor symptoms of PD (Kurth et al., 1997). Fava et al. (1999) examined the efficacy of tolcapone in treating primary major depression (i.e., depression in the absence of known neurologic dysfunction). The study included 21 patients with major depression, who received 8 weeks of tolcapone, 400 mg twice daily. There was a significant reduction of depression scores over time, and 67% of the patients reported to be much or very much improved after treatment completion. Eight patients (38%) dropped out before completing the study owing to diarrhea, elevated liver function tests, increased anxiety, or non-compliance. Whereas this preliminary study suggests that tolcapone may be useful in treating depression in PD, there are recent reports of patients who developed life-threatening hepatocellular injury during treatment, and tolcapone should not be used in patients with liver disease (Fava et al., 1999).

Di Rocco et al. (2000) examined the efficacy of S-adenosyl-methionine (SAM) in an open-label study that included 11 depressed PD patients. SAM was started at 800 mg/day in two divided doses, and titrated within a 6-week period until depression improved or a maximun dose of 3600 mg/day was achieved. Ten of the 11 patients had a significant response (defined as a decrease of at least 50% of the baseline HAM-D scores), and the only relevant side-effect was increased anxiety in two patients.

Electroconvulsive therapy

Electroconvulsive therapy (ECT) should be considered in those PD patients who do not respond to antidepressant drug treatment, whenever serious medical conditions (e.g., malnutrition, dehydration) do not allow the patient to wait for the response of psychoactive drugs, or whenever cardiovascular conditions suggest a high risk of complications with antidepressant drugs. ECT is a low-risk procedure, and cardiovascular complications rarely occur. The most frequent side-effect of ECT in elderly patients is a transitory confusional state, although the severity and duration of this confusional state is usually mild and short-lasting.

Several studies demonstrated significant mood improvement in PD patients treated with ECT. Douyon et al. (1989) used bilateral ECT to treat seven depressed PD patients, which produced a significant mood improvement in all seven patients. Moreover, there were also significant improvements in postural instability, gait, tremor, bradykinesia, and rigidity. During a 6-month follow-up period, two of these seven patients had a relapse into depression. Moellentine et al. (1998) carried out a retrospective study that compared the mood and motor outcome of 25 PD patients and 25 depressed individuals without PD, matched for age and gender, who received ECT for psychiatric indications. They found a similar marked improvement in affective symptoms (both depression and anxiety) in PD and non-PD depressed groups. Moreover, 14 of the 25 PD patients also had a transient improvement in their parkinsonian signs, and none of them had increased cognitive deficits after ECT completion, although 13 of the 25 PD patients developed a short-lasting inter-treatment delirium.

The finding that ECT may have antiparkinsonian effects on its own was replicated in several studies. Balldin et al. (1981) treated with ECT a series of nine PD patients with On–Off motor fluctuations. After an average of six treatments, there was a marked reduction of the Off time in five patients, and this benefit lasted for 4–41 weeks. The remaining four patients showed only minor or no improvement. Anderson et al. (1987) assigned 11 non-depressed PD patients with On–Off motor fluctuations to receive ECT or sham treatment (i.e., anesthesia without induction of electrical stimulation). They found that patients receiving ECT had a significant reduction in Off time compared with patients with sham treatment, and this motor improvement lasted from 2 to 6 weeks. Rasmussen and Abrams (1992) suggested that advanced age and severe disability may constitute favorable prognostic factors for an ECT mood response and also mentioned that treatment-emergent dyskinesias may occur during ECT but may respond to l-dopa dosage reduction. In most studies, no significant correlations were found between the improvement of parkinsonian signs and mood changes after ECT. Motor symptoms may respond sooner than depression, but may also relapse sooner.

Transcranial magnetic stimulation (TMS) is regularly used as a diagnostic tool for a variety of neurologic disorders (Barker et al., 1986). Several recent studies suggest that repeated TMS (rTMS) may be a useful tool in treating depression (George et al., 1997). Unlike conventional ECT, rTMS delivers a highly localized electric stimulus to a brain area using much less voltage, and no seizures are induced. Mally and Stone (1999) treated a series of 49 PD patients with rTMS and noted a significant and long-lasting improvement in motor symptoms of PD, but no information was provided about changes in depression status.

Psychotherapy

Cognitive therapy may be an adequate treatment modality for some depressed PD patients, but its efficacy has not been empirically examined. Brown and Jahanshahi (1995) suggested that key factors for the treatment of depression in PD are: "availability and quality of social supports, the types of strategies that the individual uses to cope with stress, the explanatory cognitions and perceptions of control, and attitudes and beliefs about the self." They pointed out that PD is associated with loss of job satisfaction and decrease in self-esteem. Singer (1973) carried out a survey which demonstrated that only 51% of PD males below 65 years of age were still working compared with 82% in demographic statistics, and similar figures were found for female patients (7% vs 43%, respectively). Brown and Jahanshahi (1995) pointed out that patients may become progressively reluctant to participate in social events outside the home owing to the embarrassment produced by the motor symptoms of PD, thus developing a more restricted lifestyle with "premature social aging" (Singer, 1973). Based on this evidence, Brown and Jahanshahi (1995) suggested that a psycho-therapy program for depressed PD patients should be individually "tailored" to each patient and should include other family members as well. Treatment should focus on the disabilities and handicaps produced by the illness and should be continuous throughout the course of the disease to help the patient adjust to the new circumstances imposed by the disease.

Carter et al. (1998) examined, in a series of 380 spouses of PD patients, the relationship between stage of illness and relevant caregiving variables, such as caregiver role strain, the caregiving situation, and characteristics of the caregiver. The overall finding was a significant association between advanced stage of illness and greater role strain. Hoehn and Yahr stage 2 was characterized by increasing worry, stage 3 was characterized by an increased strain in the areas of worry, tension, frustration from communication problems, direct care, role conflict, and global strain, and the last stages of the illness were characterized by a significant strain from lack of resources, economic burden, feelings of being manipulated, and mismatched expecta-tions. They also reported that the mean number of caregiving tasks doubled at stage 3, and tripled by stage 4/5. These increasing demands on caregivers across the stages of the illness were associated with negative changes in lifestyle and a decrease in caregivers' life control and predictability. The authors suggested that psycho-educational interventions and in-home res-pite care may help to reduce caregivers' strain. Aarsland et al. (1999a) assessed the emotional and social distress of caring for PD patients. They found that caregivers of PD patients suffer a substantial level of emotional distress and stress related to caregiving, and that the psychologic health of spouses was worse than in elderly controls. Depression and cognitive deficits of the patient were the most important variables associated with caregivers' stress. On the other hand, they found that stage of illness, severity of motor symptoms, and social support available to the caregivers were not related to caregiver distress.

In conclusion, several studies have demonstrated the efficacy of pharmacologic treatment in depressed PD patients. Tricyclics seem to be the most useful medications, although the high prevalence of side-effects may limit their usefulness. SSRIs are better tolerated than tricyclics but may exacerbate parkinsonian signs in some PD patients, and their efficacy has not been examined in controlled studies. ECT is a useful treatment modality for PD patients with depression that is refractory to medical treatment. The rate of response to ECT in PD is similar to the rate of response in depressed patients without PD. Finally, psychotherapeutic interventions may be tailored to each patient's needs, and may also consider strategies to reduce burden in caregivers.

Treatment of psychosis in PD

Musser and Mayada (1996) proposed a three-step treatment approach for psychosis in PD, which includes: (1) the identification of potential under-lying causes of confusional states (e.g., urinary and pulmonary infections, strokes, metabolic changes), (2) the gradual reduction of antiparkinsonian medication, and (3) the commencement of treatment with atypical anti-psychotics (i.e., drugs with a low incidence of parkinsonian side-effects at usual doses) (Figure 8.1). Wolters (1999) suggested that treatment of psychosis in PD should start with an explanation of the condition to both the patient and the caregiver, followed by a reduction of either sensory deprivation or overload, and the organization of an active day program. He stressed the importance of making a differential diagnosis between causes of psychosis, such as late-onset paraphrenia, psychosis secondary to dementia, drug-induced psychotic relapse, drug-induced acute delirium, or drug-induced (chronic) dopaminergic psychosis, since only the last of these may benefit from low-dose antipsychotics.

Factor et al. (1995b) suggested that pharmacotherapy may not be necess-ary when hallucinations are brief and intermittent, in the context of clear sensorium and normal insight, but there is consensus that neuroleptics are needed in a sizeable proportion of PD patients with psychosis (Valldeoriola et al., 1997). We will review the efficacy of those neuroleptic drugs that are most widely used in treating psychosis in PD.

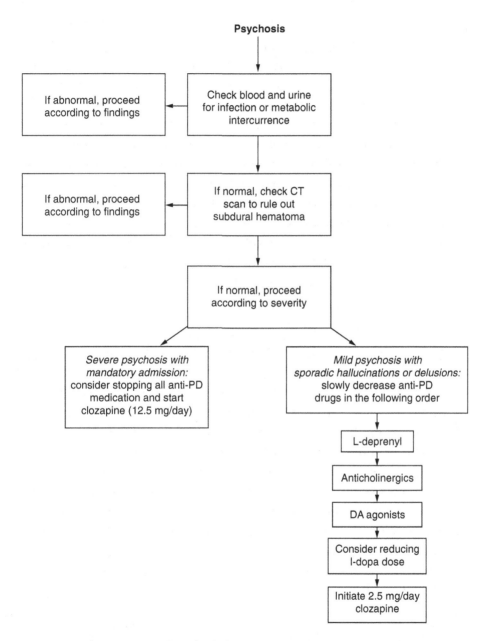

Figure 8.1. The treatment of psychosis in PD.

Clozapine

Clozapine is a dibenzodiazepine derivative with a strong affinity for dopaminergic receptors D_1, D_3, and D_4, and a lower affinity for D_2 receptors, as well as antiserotonergic, antihistaminergic, antinoradrenergic, and anticholinergic effects. There are few controlled studies of clozapine in PD, and most of them are open-label or small case series. Trosch et al. (1998) carried out a multicenter, retrospective review of clozapine in 172 consecutive PD patients with psychosis treated at four different movement disorders clinics. They found marked clinical improvements in visual and auditory hallucinations in 90% of the patients, whereas delusions improved in 90%, anxiety in 83%, depression in 60%, insomnia in 72%, and sundowning in 54%. Thirty percent of the patients had to discontinue clozapine owing to adverse events, but no cases of agranulocytosis were reported. The most frequent side-effect was daytime sedation (46% of the patients), followed by sialorrhea (11%), orthostatic hypotension (10%), memory loss (6%), and worsening parkinsonism (5%).

The Parkinson Study Group (1999) carried out a multicenter, randomized, placebo-controlled, double-blind study of clozapine for the treatment of psychosis in PD. The trial lasted for 4 weeks, and antiparkinsonian drugs were administered during the trial period at fixed doses. All doses were started at 6.25 mg and could be raised to the next level (6.25 mg more) depending on the patient's clinical response, up to 50 mg/day. Sixty PD patients with delusions and hallucinations entered the study, and 54 patients completed the study, with a mean daily dose of clozapine of 24.7 mg. There was a significant improvement from clozapine over placebo as measured with specific psychiatric scales, and 48% of the patients on clozapine were very much improved, compared with only 11% of the patients on placebo. Three patients on clozapine discontinued the study: one due to leukopenia, another due to a myocardial infarction, and a third due to sedation. Patients on clozapine showed a significant weight increment (0.7 kg) compared with the placebo group (0.1 kg), and an increased pulse rate, but no other significant side-effects associated with clozapine were reported. It is important to note that clozapine not only did not worsen motor function, but also decreased tremor. The authors found that clozapine did not impair memory and general cognition, and there was no increased incidence of anticholinergic effects or somnolence. A 12-week, prospective, open-label extension of the trial demonstrated that patients originally treated with placebo had a similar degree of improvement as the group originally treated with clozapine (Factor et al., 2001).

The French Clozapine Study Group (1999) studied 60 PD patients with no or mild dementia, who showed psychosis despite discontinuation of anticholinergic drugs or dopaminergic agonists. All patients were randomized into a 4-week, double-blind, placebo-controlled study using an initial clozapine dose of 6.25 mg/day, which was titrated over 10 days to a maximun of 50 mg/day. At the end of the study, the mean daily dose of clozapine was 36 mg. There was a significant improvement for the clozapine group compared with the placebo group, with no significant changes in MMSE or UPDRS scores. Adverse events were similar for both groups, although patients on clozapine showed more severe somnolence. None of the patients developed agranulocytosis.

Treatment with clozapine was also reported to allow patients to stay on the usual dose of l-dopa, and in some reports l-dopa dose could be increased without relapse of psychotic symptoms (Wolters et al., 1996; Ruggieri et al., 1997). Bonuccelli et al. (1997) reported a significant reduction of both resting and postural tremor under clozapine treatment, and this benefit was maintained on chronic clozapine administration. Pakkenberg and Pakkenberg (1986) reported that six out of nine PD patients treated with clozapine had a considerable improvement in tremor severity, with a marked decrease in frequency and amplitude. Friedman and Lannon (1990) used clozapine in five PD patients with tremor refractory to dopaminergic medications, with a marked improvement in one patient and moderate improvements in the other four. Jansen (1994) used clozapine in 23 PD patients who were refractory to antiparkinsonian medications, and found that 73% of the patients had an important long-lasting improvement in scores of tremor. Since most of these patients had failed trials of anticholinergics with greater anticholinergic potency than clozapine, Factor and Friedman (1997) suggested that the anti-tremor effect of clozapine may be mediated by non-cholinergic mechanisms. Other authors reported improvements in bradykinesia and gait after starting clozapine in psychotic PD patients (Friedman & Lannon, 1989; Roberts et al., 1989). Bennett et al. (1993) found a marked reduction of dyskinesias and Off time, and were also able to optimize the dose of antiparkinsonian agents without the recurrence of psychotic symptoms. They suggested that the antidyskinetic effect of clozapine may be related to D_1-antagonist activity in the nigrostriatal dopamine system. Clozapine also has an important sleep-inducing effect, which may benefit patients with insomnia (Factor & Brown, 1992). Some reports suggest that clozapine may be less effective in PD patients with dementia, but this was not confirmed (see Factor et al., 1995b, for a review).

There is no general agreement as to the length of clozapine therapy in PD, but Friedman (1995) suggested that patients should be on full dosage of clozapine for at least 1 month following the resolution of psychotic symptoms, after which the dose should be slowly tapered off. There are few long-term prospective studies of clozapine treatment for psychosis in PD. Some studies suggest that the efficacy of clozapine declines with time, whereas others found continuous benefit. Wagner et al. (1996) reported a retrospective chart review of 49 PD patients with psychotic symptoms who were treated with clozapine for up to 18 months. They found that 92% of the patients had a positive response to clozapine at some point during treatment, but some patients who were initially non-responders became responders, and vice versa, suggesting that some patients may develop tolerance to clozapine. Wagner et al. (1996) also found a high rate of relapse for those patients who discontinued treatment, suggesting that some patients may require continued clozapine therapy.

One of the benefits of clozapine is its high efficacy and lack of impact on parkinsonian signs, provided that doses of about 100 mg/day are not exceeded (doses of 250 mg/day were found to exacerbate parkinsonism). The most frequent side-effects of clozapine are sedation, orthostatic hypotension, tachycardia, weight gain, hypothermia, and drooling. Since orthostatic hypotension is a frequent problem in PD patients, blood pressure should be measured both in recumbent and standing positions on a daily basis during the first week of treatment (Pinter & Helscher 1993). Clozapine was also reported to induce seizures in about 1% of patients with schizophrenia, and should be used cautiously in PD patients with a history of epilepsy (Auzou et al., 1996). The most serious side-effect of clozapine is agranulocytosis, which is not dose-related, and occurs in about 1–2% of schizophrenic patients. Weekly blood counts are mandatory, and should include differential counts, since neutropenia may occur while the white-cell count remains stable. Treatment should be stopped whenever the white cell count is less than 3000 cells per cubic millimeter or whenever absolute neutrophil counts are less than 1500 cells per cubic millimeter. Clozapine should definitely be discontinued with white blood counts of less than 2000 cells per cubic millimeter and neutrophil counts of less than 1000 cells per cubic millimeter. This drug should be avoided in patients with a history of drug-related blood dyscrasias or in patients with a baseline white cell count of less than 3000 cells per cubic millimeter or a neutrophil count of less than 1500 cells per cubic millimeter (Auzou et al., 1996).

Risperidone

Risperidone is an atypical antipsychotic drug with potent serotonin 5-HT_2 and weak dopamine D_2 receptor antagonist properties. It also has high α-adrenergic and histamine, but low muscarinic, blockade potency. The efficacy of risperidone in treating PD psychosis was examined in a few studies. Meco et al. (1997) treated 10 PD patients with psychosis using risperidone with a starting dose of 0.25 mg at bedtime, which was increased until control of psychosis was achieved or side-effects appeared. Using a dose of risperidone ranging from 0.25 mg/day to 1.25 mg/day, they found a significant improvement in 9 out of 10 patients. There was no significant increment in parkinsonian signs, although two patients had to discontinue risperidone due to worsening of parkinsonism, and two other patients had to be hospitalized due to confusion and psychomotor agitation. Less important side-effects were sialorrhea, and drowsiness. During the 24-week treatment period there was also a significant drop in MMSE scores, which did not improve following discontinuation of risperidone treatment. Workman et al. (1997) treated nine psychotic and demented PD patients with risperidone with a mean dose of 1.9 mg/day (range: 1–3 mg/day). They found a significant improvement in psychotic symptoms and an improvement in global functioning, without significant side-effects. Leopold (2000) used risperidone (0.5–1.5 mg/day) in a series of 35 PD patients with hallucinations. Twenty-three patients (59%) had a complete or partial remission of hallucinations, six patients had no improvement, and six patients had worsening of parkinsonism. Mohr et al. (2000) examined the tolerability, safety, and efficacy of risperidone in an open-label study that included 17 patients with PD and psychosis. They found a fast and effective antipsychotic action of risperidone at low doses (0.5–1.0 mg/day). On the other hand, adverse effects such as hypokinesia and somnolence were quite frequent.

Ellis et al. (2000) carried out a randomized, double-blind comparison trial of clozapine and risperidone in 10 PD patients with psychosis. They found both drugs to have similar efficacy in improving psychosis. One patient in each group developed an important worsening of parkinsonian signs, and one patient on clozapine developed neutropenia. UPDRS scores worsened in the risperidone group and showed some improvement in the clozapine group, but the sample size was too small to allow definite conclusions.

Olanzapine

Olanzapine is an atypical antipsychotic with a high affinity for dopaminergic and serotonergic receptors. Wolters et al. (1996) examined the efficacy of olanzapine in an open-label drug trial that included 15 PD patients with psychosis. Olanzapine produced a significant clinical improvement in 14 patients, which was evident within 2–5 weeks after starting treatment. Moreover, all 14 patients could tolerate an increase in l-dopa doses, with a concomitant improvement in motor symptoms and no psychiatric relapse. The final daily dosage of olanzapine ranged from 2 mg/day to 15 mg/day, and neither major nor minor side-effects were reported. However, Jimenez-Jimenez et al. (1998) reported two PD patients who were treated with a low dose of olanzapine (5 mg/day) and who developed more severe bradykinesia and rigidity. Both patients improved after clozapine was substituted for olanzapine. Manson et al. (2000) reported olanzapine as reducing the severity of dyskinesias, but increasing parkinsonian signs and Off time.

Aarsland et al. (1999b) examined the efficacy of olanzapine in an open-label, 8-week trial that included 21 PD patients with psychosis. The starting dose of olanzapine was 5 mg/day, but due to frequent side-effects, the starting dose was reduced to 2.5 mg/day. Twelve out of 15 patients who completed 8 weeks of treatment had a marked improvement, with significant declines in scores of delusions, hallucinations, and agitation. At week 8, 14 of the 15 patients were on 2.5 mg/day or 5 mg/day. There were no significant changes in parkinsonian signs or cognitive functioning during the treatment period. Most frequent side-effects were concentration difficulties, memory impairment, increased sleep duration, and dryness of mouth.

Friedman (1998) reported 19 patients with parkinsonism due to Lewy body disease ($n=3$), PD ($n=10$), neuroleptic-induced parkinsonism ($n=3$), or related disorders ($n=3$), who participated in an open-label study with olanzapine. They found that in PD patients, olanzapine, even at low doses, frequently produced an increase in parkinsonism, and that only five of the nine PD patients benefited from this drug. Friedman et al. (1998) also examined whether PD patients on clozapine could be switched to olanzapine, given that the former drug requires weekly blood tests, whereas olanzapine is devoid of this requirement. The study involved 12 PD patients who were psychiatrically stable on clozapine but who were interested in stopping their weekly blood tests. The trial started by adding olanzapine 2.5 mg at bedtime, then slowly tapering off the clozapine (about 1.25 mg each week) as the dose of olanzapine was increased (about 2.5 mg each time). This process lasted for 1–4 weeks. The main finding was that, in most cases, olanzapine had to be stopped because of increased parkinsonism, and that only three of the 12 patients decided to continue on olanzapine.

Goetz et al. (2000) carried out a randomized, double-blind comparison trial of clozapine and olanzapine in a series of 15 PD patients with hallucinations. They found clozapine to be more effective than olanzapine in treating the hallucinations. Moreover, olanzapine produced a significant increment in the severity of parkinsonian signs, whereas no significant changes in motor function were found in the clozapine group. The authors interpreted their findings as strongly in support of clozapine (compared with olanzapine) in PD patients.

Other antipsychotics

Quetiapine is another atypical antipsychotic, with a higher affinity for serotonin 5-HT$_2$ than dopamine D$_1$ or D$_2$ receptors. Parsa and Bastani (1998) treated two psychotic PD patients with quetiapine in a 5-week, open-label, clinical trial. Both patients had a successful clinical response without increment in parkinsonian signs or other side-effects. Targum and Abbott (2000) reported good efficacy of quetiapine in controlling hallucinations, but less efficacy in controlling delusions. Juncos et al. (2000) carried out a 24-week, open-label trial with quetiapine in a series of 29 PD patients with psychosis who had failed previous treatments with clozapine, risperidone, or olanzapine. They found a 30% improvement in their endpoint measure (the Brief Psychiatric Rating Scale). No important side-effects were reported, and there were no significant changes in the motor section of the UPDRS. Dewey and O'Suilleabhain (2000) reported a retrospective study of 84 PD patients with psychosis who were given quetiapine. Nine patients were switched to clozapine owing to inadequate efficacy of quetiapine, and eight of them had good control of psychosis. Fourteen patients were lost to follow-up. Of the remaining 61 patients, 40 remained on quetiapine with good control of hallucinations. The most common side-effect of quetiapine was sedation, but modification of dopaminergic therapy was not necessary.

Fernandez et al. (1999) reported that only three out of eight PD patients could be successfully switched from clozapine to quetiapine. In a subsequent study that included 15 new patients, they used a slower titration schedule of quetiapine, and a wider overlap period of clozapine and quetiapine (Fernandez et al., 2000). They found that 12 of the patients were able to switch to quetiapine without loss of antipsychotic effect or worsening of cognitive or motor functions. At 12-month follow-up, nine of the 12 patients that switched successfully to quetiapine remained without psychosis, whereas three patients had to switch back to clozapine owing to increased parkinsonism.

Ondansetron is a selective 5-HT$_3$ receptor antagonist used as an antiemetic in cancer patients receiving chemotherapy (Marty et al., 1990). Zoldan et al. (1995) treated, with this drug, a series of 16 PD patients with 6–60 months of psychosis, who continued to receive their optimal antiparkinsonian therapy throughout the trial. Fifteen of the 16 patients improved upon treatment with ondansetron, with marked remissions of visual hallucinations and paranoid delusions. The drug was well tolerated, and side-effects were minor (e.g.,constipation and mild headaches). Eichorn et al. (1996) treated, with ondansetron, a series of seven PD patients with hallucinations, paranoid delusions, and confusion. Ondansetron was administered orally at a daily dosage of 8–24 mg, without change in antiparkinsonian medications. Five of the seven patients failed to respond to ondansetron; two had been on the highest dose of 24 mg/day for at least 2 weeks, whereas the other three patients had been on 12 mg/day for the same period. Two patients had a good therapeutic response, but in one of them the antipsychotic effect lasted for only 7 weeks.

Other treatments for psychosis

ECT may be useful in treating psychosis in PD, but no controlled studies of this technique have been carried out until now. Hurwitz et al. (1988) carried out ECT in two psychotic PD patients, who showed great clinical improvement that lasted for about 5 months. Factor et al. (1995a) reported significant improvements with ECT in a small group of psychotic PD patients, but improvements were transient and required long-term treatment with clozapine.

In conclusion, recent empirical data demonstrated an important role for atypical antipsychotics in the treatment of drug-induced psychosis in PD. Clozapine is considered to be the drug of choice, since it provides potent antipsychotic efficacy together with anti-tremor effect and a low profile of side-effects (Friedman & Factor, 2000). The consensus is that more than 80% of psychotic PD patients may improve upon treatment with clozapine (Wolters, 1999). This effect is achieved with clozapine doses that are considerably lower than the ones used to treat schizophrenia: in PD this drug is usually started at 6.25 mg/day or 12.5 mg/day and progressively increased until the resolution of psychotic symptoms (usually with less than 100 mg/day). No deaths related to granulocytopenia have been reported until now among PD patients. Quetiapine and olanzapine were reported to have a similar efficacy and profile of side-effects, and may be an option to clozapine. They are easier to use as they do not require weekly blood cell counts. Risperidone is more poorly tolerated than the other atypical antipsychotics and may be a third treatment option, whereas ondansetron did not demonstrate a higher efficacy than the atypical antipsychotics.

General conclusions

The ultimate role of the different types of antidepressant medications in PD remains to be empirically determined. Tom and Cummings (1998) suggested an algorithmic approach to the treatment of depression in PD based on the following recommendations: each antidepressant should have at least a 6-week trial at the maximum tolerated therapeutic range; the adverse effect profile of SSRIs may be more favorable than tricyclic antidepressants for PD patients and should be preferred; and once the patient becomes euthymic, the medication should be continued for at least 6 months or longer. Finally, they also advised against combining selegiline with SSRIs or tricyclic antidepressants, as there is an increased risk of these combinations producing a "serotonin syndrome." ECT was reported to be useful among PD patients with drug-refractory depressions, with the added benefit of a transient improvement in parkinsonian signs. Given the impact of disabilities in ADLs and the concomitant strain in marital relationships, structured psychologic interventions may benefit a subgroup of highly motivated PD patients. Treatment of PD patients with psychosis should start by identifying potential causes for the behavioral change, and adjusting antiparkinsonian medication, if possible. The actual consensus is that atypical antipsychotics such as clozapine, olanzapine, and quetiapine may be the most adequate drugs in treating psychosis in PD, but controlled studies on the efficacy of some of these compounds are still needed.

Appendix: scales for clinical assessment

A wide variety of methods are used to assess PD, such as self-reports of parkinsonian symptoms, examiner-rated assessments, and sophisticated quantitative physiologic measurements of parkinsonian signs. Ideally, a rating scale for PD should: (1) be easy to use, (2) require a short time to administer, (3) be both valid and reliable, and (4) be predictive of further impairment. The most frequently used scales in PD are listed in the following pages.

A.1 Unified Parkinson's disease rating scale (UPDRS) (adapted from Langston et al., 1992)

This scale assesses the cardinal features of PD, the complications of treatment, and the impact of treatment on patients' mood, mentation, behavior, and activities of daily life. The UPDRS evaluates four components: (1) Mentation behavior and mood, (2) activities of daily living, (3) motor examination, and (4) complications of therapy. Scores range from 0 (normal) to 199 (worst clinical state).

I. Mentation, behavior, mood
1   **Intellectual impairment**

    0   None

    1   Mild (consistent forgetfulness with partial recollection of events with no difficulties)

    2   Moderate memory loss with disorientation and moderate difficulty in handling complex problems

    3   Severe memory loss with disorientation in time and often place; severe impairment with problems

    4   Severe memory loss with orientations only to person; unable to make judgments or solve problems

2   Thought disorder

0   None

1   Vivid dreaming

2   "Benign" hallucination with insight retained

3   Occasional to frequent hallucinations or delusions without insight, which could interfere with daily activities

3   Depression

0   None

1   Periods of sadness or guilt greater than normal; never sustained for more than a few days or a week

2   Sustained depression for 1 week

3   Vegetative symptoms (insomnia, anorexia, abulia, weight loss)

4   Vegetative symptoms with suicide ideation

4   Motivation/initiative

0   Normal

1   Less assertive than usual, more passive

2   Loss of initiative or disinterest in elective (non-routine) activities

3   Loss of initiative or disinterest in day-to-day (routine) activities

4   Withdrawn, complete loss of motivation

II. Activities of daily living (specify for "On/Off")

5   Speech

0   Normal

1   Mildly affected; no difficulty in being understood

2   Moderately affected; may be asked to repeat

3   Severely affected, frequently asked to repeat

4   Unintelligible most of the time

6   Salivation

0   Normal

1   Slight but noticeable increase; may have night-time drooling

2   Moderately excessive saliva; may have minimal drooling

3   Marked drooling

7   Swallowing

0   Normal

1   Rare choking
2   Occasional choking
3   Requires soft food
4   Requires nasogastric or gastric tube

8   Handwriting

0   Normal
1   Slightly small or slow
2   All words small but legible
3   Severely affected; not all words legible
4   Most words illegible

9   Cutting food, handling utensils

0   Normal
1   Somewhat slow and clumsy but no help needed
2   Can cut most foods but some help needed
3   Food must be cut but can feed self
4   Needs to be fed

10   Dressing

0   Normal
1   Somewhat slow but no help needed
2   Occasional help with buttons or arms in sleeves
3   Considerable help needed but can do some things alone
4   Helpless

11   Hygiene

0   Normal
1   Somewhat slow but no help needed
2   Needs help with shower or bath or very slow in hygienic care
3   Requires help for washing, brushing teeth, going to bathroom
4   Helpless

12   Turning in bed and adjusting bed clothes

0   Normal
1   Somewhat slow but no help needed
2   Can turn alone or adjust sheets but with great difficulty
3   Can initiate but not turn or adjust alone
4   Helpless

13   Falling (unrelated to freezing)

0   None
1   Rare falls
2   Occasional falls; fewer than one per day
3   Average of one fall per day
4   Falls more than once daily

14   Freezing when walking

0   None
1   Rare freezing; may have start hesitation
2   Occasional falls from freezing
3   Frequent freezing; occasional falls
4   Frequent falls from freezing

15   Walking

0   Normal
1   Mild difficulty; may drag legs or decrease arm swing
2   Moderate difficulty; requires no assistance
3   Severe disturbance; requires assistance
4   Cannot walk at all, even with assistance

16   Tremor

0   Absent
1   Slight and infrequent; not bothersome to patient
2   Moderate; bothersome to patient
3   Severe; interferes with many activities
4   Marked; interferes with many activities

17   Sensory complaints related to parkinsonism

0   None
1   Occasionally has numbness, tingling, and mild aching
2   Frequent but not distressing complaints
3   Frequent painful sensation
4   Excruciating pain

III. Motor examination

18   Speech

0   Normal

1   Slight loss of expression, diction, and volume
2   Monotone; slurred but understandable; moderately impaired
3   Markedly impaired; difficult to understand
4   Unintelligible

19   Facial expression

0   Normal
1   Slight hypomimia; could be poker-faced
2   Slight but definite abnormal diminution in expression
3   Moderate hypomimia; lips parted some of time
4   Masked or fixed face; lips parted one-quarter inch (6 mm) or more with complete loss of expression

20   Tremor at rest

Face

0   Absent
1   Slight and infrequent
2   Mild and present most of the time
3   Moderate and present most of the time
4   Marked and present most of the time

Right upper extremity (RUE)

0   Absent
1   Slight and infrequent
2   Mild and present most of the time
3   Moderate and present most of the time
4   Marked and present most of the time

Left upper extremity (LUE)

0   Absent
1   Slight and infrequent
2   Mild and present most of the time
3   Moderate and present most of the time
4   Marked and present most of the time

Right lower extremity (RLE)

0   Absent
1   Slight and infrequent
2   Mild and present most of the time
3   Moderate and present most of the time
4   Marked and present most of the time

Left lower extremity (LLE)

0   Absent
1   Slight and infrequent
2   Mild and present most of the time
3   Moderate and present most of the time
4   Marked and present most of the time

21   Action or postural tremor

RUE

0   Absent
1   Slight; present with action
2   Moderate; present with action
3   Moderate; present with action and posture holding
4   Marked; interferes with feeding

LUE

0   Absent
1   Slight; present with action
2   Moderate; present with action
3   Moderate; present with action and posture holding
4   Marked; interferes with feeding

22   Rigidity

Neck

0   Absent
1   Slight or only with activation
2   Mild to moderate
3   Marked but with full range of motion
4   Severe

RUE

0   Absent
1   Slight or only with activation
2   Mild to moderate
3   Marked but with full range of motion
4   Severe

LUE

0   Absent
1   Slight or only with activation

2   Mild to moderate
3   Marked but with full range of motion
4   Severe

RLE

0   Absent
1   Slight or only with activation
2   Mild to moderate
3   Marked but with full range of motion
4   Severe

LLE

0   Absent
1   Slight or only with activation
2   Mild to moderate
3   Marked but with full range of motion
4   Severe

23   Finger taps
Right

0   Normal
1   Mild slowing; reduction in amplitude; or both
2   Moderately impaired; definite and early fatiguing; may have occasional arrests
3   Severely impaired; frequent hesitations and arrests
4   Can barely perform

Left

0   Normal
1   Mild slowing; reduction in amplitude; or both
2   Moderately impaired; definite and early fatiguing; may have occasional arrests
3   Severely impaired; frequent hesitations and arrests
4   Can barely perform

24   Hand movements (open and close hands in rapid succession)
Right

0   Normal
1   Mild slowing; reduction in amplitude; or both
2   Moderately impaired; definite and early fatiguing; may have occasional arrests

3   Severely impaired; frequent hesitations and arrests
4   Can barely perform

Left

0   Normal
1   Mild slowing; reduction in amplitude; or both
2   Moderately impaired; definite and early fatiguing; may have occasional arrests
3   Severely impaired; frequent hesitations and arrests
4   Can barely perform

25   Rapid alternating movements (pronate and supinate hands)

Right

0   Normal
1   Mild slowing; reduction in amplitude; or both
2   Moderately impaired; definite and early fatiguing; may have occasional arrests
3   Severely impaired; frequent hesitations and arrests
5   Can barely perform

Left

0   Normal
1   Mild slowing; reduction in amplitude; or both
2   Moderately impaired; definite and early fatiguing; may have occasional arrests
3   Severely impaired; frequent hesitations and arrests
4   Can barely perform

26   Leg agility (tap heel on ground: amplitude should be 3"/7.5 cm)

Right

0   Normal
1   Mild slowing; reduction in amplitude; or both
2   Moderately impaired; definite and early fatiguing; may have occasional arrests
3   Severely impaired; frequent hesitations and arrests
4   Can barely perform

Left

0   Normal
1   Mild slowing; reduction in amplitude; or both
2   Moderately impaired; definite and early fatiguing; may have occasional arrests
3   Severely impaired; frequent hesitations and arrests
4   Can barely perform

27   Rising from chair (patient rises with arms folded across chest)
0   Normal
1   Slow; may need more than one attempt
2   Pushes self up from arms or seat
3   Tends to fall back; may need multiple attempts but can rise without help
4   Unable to rise without help

28   Posture
0   Normal erect
1   Slightly stooped; could be normal for older person
2   Definitely abnormal; moderately stooped; may lean to one side
3   Severely stooped with kyphosis
4   Marked flexion with extreme abnormality of posture

29   Gait
0   Normal
1   Walks slowly; may shuffle with short steps; no festination or propulsion
2   Walks with difficulty; little or no assistance needed; some festination; short steps
      or propulsion
3   Severe disturbance; frequent assistance needed
4   Cannot walk

30   Postural stability (retropulsion test)
0   Normal
1   Recovers unaided
2   Would fall if not caught
3   Falls spontaneously
4   Unable to stand

31   Body bradykinesia and hypokinesia
0   None
1   Minimal slowness; could be normal; deliberate character
2   Mild slowness and poverty of movement; definitely abnormal; decreased ampli-
      tude of movement
3   Moderate slowness; poverty; small amplitude of movement
4   Marked slowness; poverty; small amplitude of movement

IV. Complications of therapy (during the previous week)

DYSKINESIAS

32   **Duration: What proportion of the waking day are dyskinesias present (medical history)?**

0   None
1   1–25% of day
2   26–50% of day
3   51–75% of day
4   76–100% of day

33   **Disability: How disabling are the dyskinesias (medical history, may be modified by office examination)?**

0   Not disabling
1   Mildly disabling
2   Moderately disabling
3   Severely disabling
4   Completely disabling

34   **Painful dyskinesias: How painful are the dyskinesias?**

0   Not painful
1   Slightly
2   Moderately
3   Markedly
4   Severely

35   **Presence of early morning dystonia (medical history)**

0   No
1   Yes

CLINICAL FLUCTUATIONS

36   **"Off" periods: Are any predictable as to timing after a dose of medication?**

0   No
1   Yes

37   **"Off" periods: Are any unpredictable as to timing after a dose of medication?**

0   No
1   Yes

38   "Off" periods: Do any come on suddenly (e.g., over a few seconds)?

0   No
1   Yes

39   "Off" periods: What proportion of the waking day is the patient "Off" on average?

0   None
1   1–25% of day
2   26–50% of day
3   51–75% of day
4   76–100% of day

OTHER COMPLICATIONS

40   Does the patient have anorexia, nausea, or vomiting?

0   No
1   Yes

41   Does the patient have any sleep disturbances (e.g., insomnia or hypersomnolence)?

0   No
1   Yes

42   Does the patient have symptomatic orthostasis?

0   No
1   Yes

A.2 Dyskinesia rating scale (adapted from Goetz et al., 1994)

This scale allows the examiner to rate the severity and duration of involuntary movements.

Severity

0   Absent
1   Minimal severity; patient is not aware of dyskinesia
2   Patient is conscious of the presence of dyskinesias, but there is no interference with voluntary motor acts (or completion of the motor acts of the rated task)
3   Dyskinesias may impair voluntary movements, but the patient is normally

capable of undertaking most motor tasks (or completing the motor acts of the
rated task)

4   Intense interference with motor control (or completion of the motor acts of the
rated task); daily life activities are greatly limited

5   Violent dyskinesias, incompatible with any motor task

Duration

0   Absent

1   Present only when carrying out motor tasks

2   Present for 25–50% of waking hours

3   Present for 51–75% of waking hours

4   Present for 76–99% of waking hours

5   Continuous throughout the day: 100%

A.3 Schwab and England rating scale (adapted from Lang, 1990)

The Schwab and England activities of daily living scale assigns a value in increments of
10%, from 100% (totally normal) to 0% (total impairment, bedridden, loss of
vegetative functions). This scale may be rated by an examiner or by the patient
him-/herself

Schwab and England activities of daily living scale

100%   Completely independent; able to do all chores without slowness, difficulty,
or impairment

90%   Completely independent; able to do all chores with slowness, difficulty or
impairment; may take twice as long as usual

80%   Independent in most chores; takes twice as long as usual; conscious of
difficulty and slowing

70%   Not completely independent; more difficulty with chores; takes three to
four times as long as usual for some chores; may take large part of day for
chores

60%   Some dependence; can do most chores but very slowly and with much
effort; errors, some impossible

50%   More dependent; needs help with one-half of chores; difficulty with
everything

40%   Very dependent; can assist with all chores but can do few of them alone

30%	With effort can occasionally do a few chores alone or begin alone; much help needed
20%	Can do nothing alone; can give some slight help with some chores; severe invalid
10%	Totally dependent; helpless
0%	Vegetative functions such as swallowing and bladder and bowel function are not present; bedridden

A.4 Webster rating scale for parkinsonism (adapted from Webster, 1968)

This scale is frequently used to assess the severity of parkinsonism, and has also been used in patients with primary psychiatric illnesses. There is a close correlation between UPDRS motor scores and total scores on this scale (Nouzeilles & Merello, 1997).

1   Bradykinesia of hands

0	No involvement
1	Detectable slowness
2	Moderate slowness
3	Severe slowness; unable to write or button clothes

2   Rigidity

0	None detectable
1	Mild rigidity detectable only on activation
2	Moderate rigidity detectable at rest
3	Severe resting rigidity

3   Posture

0	Normal posture; head flexed forward less than 10 cm (4″)
1	Beginning poker spine; head flexed forwards
2	One or both arms flexed but still below waist
3	Simian posture

4   Upper extremity swing

| 0 | Both arms swing well |
| 1 | One arm definitely decreased in degree of swing |

2   One arm fails to swing
3   Both arms fail to swing

5   Gait

0   Steps out well with 18″–30″ (45.5–76 cm)
1   Stride 18″–30″; strikes one heel; takes several steps to turn
2   Stride 6″–12″ (15–30.5 cm); both heels strike floor forcefully
3   Shuffling gait and/or propulsion and intermittent freezing

6   Tremor

0   No detectable tremor
1   Mild fine-amplitude tremor; may be asymptomatic
2   Severe but not constant tremor; patient retains control of hands
3   Severe and constant tremor; writing and feeding are impossible

7   Facies

0   Normal; full animation; no stare
1   Detectable immobility
2   Moderate immobility; drooling may be present
3   Frozen facies; mouth open; drooling may be severe

8   Seborrhea

0   None
1   Increased perspiration; secretion remains thin
2   Obvious oiliness; secretion much thicker
3   Marked seborrhea; entire face and head covered by thick secretion

9   Speech

0   Clear; loud; resonant; easily understood
1   Beginning of hoarseness with loss of inflection and resonance; good volume and still easily understood
2   Moderate hoarseness and weakness; beginning of dysarthria; hesitancy; stuttering; difficult to understand
3   Marked harshness and weakness; very difficult to hear and understand

10   Self-care

0   No impairment
1   Still provides full self-care but rate of dressing impeded
2   Requires help in certain critical areas, such as turning in bed, rising from chairs, etc.; very slow in performing most activities but manages by taking a lot of time
3   Continuously disabled; unable to dress, feed himself, or walk alone

A.5 Parkinson psychosis rating scale (PPRS) (adapted from Friedberg et al., 1998)

This scale was designed to assess the severity of psychotic symptoms in patients with PD. The scale is administered by the clinician and consists of six items, each rated from 1 (no symptoms) to 4 (extreme symptoms); total scores range from 6 to 24 points.

1   Visual hallucinations

1   Absent
2   Mild: occasional; complete or partial insight; non-threatening
3   Moderate: frequent; absence of full insight; can be convinced; may be threatening
4   Severe: persistent hallucinations; no insight, associated with heightened emotional tone, agitation, and aggression

2   Illusions and misidentification of persons

1   Absent
2   Mild: occurring infrequently
3   Moderate: occurring very often
4   Severe: occurring persistently

3   Paranoid ideation (persecutory and/or jealous type)

1   Absent
2   Mild: associated with suspiciousness
3   Moderate: associated with tension and excitement
4   Severe: accusations of family members, aggression, and/or lack of cooperation (i.e., refusal to eat and/or take medication)

4   Sleep disturbances

1   Absent
2   Mild: associated with anxiety
3   Moderate: night terrors with recurrent awakening and feelings of danger
4   Severe: nightmares with recurrent awakening, associated with agitation and confusion

5   Confusion

1   Absent
2   Mild: disorientation in time/place/person
3   Moderate: confusion combined with impaired attention/concentration/registration/recall/interruption of goal-directed actions
4   Severe: very confused with or without delirium

6   Sexual preoccupation

1   Absent
2   Mild: thoughts, dreams, worry about sexual competence
3   Moderate: increased demand for sexual activity
4   Severe: violent sexual impulsiveness

SEVERITY RATING OF PARKINSONIAN PSYCHOSIS BY PPRS:

8–12   Mild
13–18   Moderate
19–24   Severe

A.6 Apathy rating scale (adapted from Starkstein et al., 1995)

This scale has proved to be both valid and reliable in rating the severity of apathy in PD. Each question has four possible answers, which are scored from 0 to 3. Thus, the apathy rating scale scores range from 0 to 42 points, and higher scores indicate more severe apathy.

Questions	Not at all	Slightly	Moderately	A lot
Are you interested in learning new things?				
Does anything interest you?				
Are you concerned about your condition?				
Do you put much effort into things?				
Are you always looking for something to do?				
Do you have plans and goals for the future?				
Do you have motivation?				
Do you have the energy for daily activities?				
Does someone have to tell you what to do each day?				
Are you indifferent to things?				
Are you unconcerned with many things?				
Do you need a push to get started on things?				
Are you neither happy nor sad, just in between?				
Would you consider yourself apathetic?				

Note: For questions 1–8, the scoring system is as follows: not at all = 3 points; slightly = 2 points; moderately = 1 point; a lot = 0 points. For questions 9–14, the scoring system is as follows: not at all = 0 points; slightly = 1 point; moderately = 2 points; a lot = 3 points.

A.7 EUROQOL rating scale (adapted from Schrag et al., 2000)

The European Quality of Life (EUROQOL) scale is a self-assessment scale that evaluates the impact of the illness on patients' lives.

Mobility

1   No problems in walking
2   Unable to walk without a stick, crutch, or walking frame
3   Confined to bed

Self-care

1   No problems with self-care
2   Unable to dress self
3   Unable to feed self

Main activity

1   Able to perform main activity (e.g., work, study, housework)
2   Unable to perform main activity

Social relationship

1   Able to pursue family and leisure activities
2   Unable to pursue family and leisure activities

Pain

1   No pain or discomfort
2   Moderate pain or discomfort
3   Extreme pain or discomfort

Mood

1   Not anxious or depressed
2   Anxious or depressed

References

Chapter 2

Acton, P.D., & Mozley, D. (2000). Single photon emission tomography imaging in parkinsonian disorders: a review. *Behavioural Neurology*, **12**, 11–27.

Agamanolis, D.P., & Greenstein, J.I. (1979). Ataxia-telangiectasia. Report of a case with Lewy bodies and vascular abnormalities within cerebral tissue. *Journal of Neuropathology and Experimental Neurology*, **38**, 475–89.

Arnulf, I., Bejjani, B.P., Garma, L., et al. (2000). Improvement of sleep architecture in PD with subthalamic nucleus stimulation. *Neurology*, **55**, 1732–4.

Barbeau, A., & Roy, M. (1982). Familial subsets in idiopathic Parkinson's disease. *Canadian Journal of Neurological Sciences*, **11**, 144–50.

Becker, G., & Berg, D. (2001). Neuroimaging in basal ganglia disorders: perspectives for transcranial ultrasound. *Movement Disorders*, **16**, 23–32.

Bedard, P.J., Gómez Mansilla, B., Blanchette, P., et al. (1997). Dopamine agonists as first line therapy of parkinsonism in MPTP monkeys: In *Beyond the Decade of the Brain*, ed. C.W. Olanow & J.A. Obeso, pp. 101–13. Kent: Wells Medical Limited.

Benabid, A.L., Pollak, P., Gervason, C.L., et al. (1991). Long-term suppression of tremor by stimulation of the ventral intermediate thalamic nucleus. *Lancet*, **337**, 403–6.

Ben-Shlomo, Y., Churchyard, A., & Head, J. (1998). Investigation by Parkinson's Disease Research Group of United Kingdom into excess mortality seen with combined levodopa and selegiline treatment inpatients with early mild Parkinson's disease: further results of randomized trial and confidential inquiry. *British Medical Journal*, **316**, 1191–6.

Bonifati, V., Fabrizio, E., Cipriani, R., et al. (1994). Buspirone in levodopa-induced dyskinesia. *Clinical Neuropharmacology*, **17**, 73–82.

Bower, J.H., Maraganore, D.M., McDonnell, S.K., & Rocca, W.A. (2000). Influence of strict, intermediate, and broad diagnostic criteria on the age-and-sex-specific incidence of Parkinson's disease. *Movement Disorders*, **15**, 819–25.

Brewis, M., Poskanzer, D.C., Rolland, C., et al. (1966). Neurological disease in an English city. *Acta Neurologica Scandinavica*, **42**, 1–89.

Bromocriptine Research Group (1989). Bromocriptine in Parkinson's disease: a double-blind study comparing "low-slow" and "high-fast" introductory dosage regimens in de novo patients. *Journal of Neurology, Neurosurgery and Psychiatry*, **52**, 77–82.

Bronstein, J.M., DeSalles, A., & DeLong, M.R. (1999). Stereotactic pallidotomy in the treatment of Parkinson disease. *Archives of Neurology*, **56**, 1064–9.

Currie, L.J., Bennett, J.P., Harrison, M.B., et al. (1997). Clinical correlates of sleep benefit in Parkinson's disease. *Neurology*, **48**, 1115–17.

Dogali, M., Fazzini, E., Kolodny, E., et al. (1995). Stereotactic ventral pallidotomy for Parkinson's disease. *Neurology*, **45**, 753–61.

Donnan, P.T., Steinke, D.T., Stubbings, C., Davey, P.G., & MacDonald, T.M. (2000). Selegiline and mortality in subjects with Parkinson's disease: a longitudinal community study. *Neurology*, **55**, 1785–9.

Dujardin, K., Krystkowiak, P., Defebvre, L., Blond, S., & Destée A. (2000). A case of severe dysexecutive syndrome consecutive to chronic bilateral pallidal stimulation. *Neuropsychologia*, **38**, 1305–15.

Duvoisin, R.C. (1984). Is Parkinson's disease acquired or inherited? *Canadian Journal of Neurological Sciences*, **11**, 151–5.

Fager, C.A. (1963). Evaluation of thalamic and subthalamic surgical lesions in the alleviation of Parkinson's disease. *Journal of Neurosurgery*, **28**, 145–9.

Fine, J., Jan Duff, R.N., Chien, R., Hutchinson, W., Lozano, A.M., & Lang, A.E. (2000). Long-term follow-up of unilateral pallidotomy in advanced Parkinson's disease. *New England Journal of Medicine*, **342**, 1708–14.

Foley, P., & Riederer, P. (2000). Influence of neurotoxins and oxidative stress on the onset and progression of Parkinson's disease. *Journal of Neurology*, **247**, 82–94.

Forno, L.S. (1987). The Lewy body in parkinson's disease. *Advances in Neurology*, **45**, 35–43.

Frankel, J.P., Lees, A.J., Kempster, P.A., & Stern, G.M. (1990). Subcutaneous apomorphine in the treatment of Parkinson's disease. *Journal of Neurology, Neurosurgery and Psychiatry*, **53**, 96–101.

Galvez-Jimenez, N., Lozano, A., Tasker, R., Duff, J., Hutchinson, W., & Lang, A.E. (1998). Pallidal stimulation in Parkinson's disease patients with a prior unilateral pallidotomy. *Canadian Journal of Neurological Sciences*, **25**, 300–5.

Garnett, E.S., Firnau, G., Nahmias, C. (1983). Dopamine visualized in the basal ganglia of living man. *Nature*, **305**, 137–8.

Ghika, J., Villemure, J.G., Fankhauser, H., Favre, J., Assal, G., & Ghika-Schmid, F. (1998). Efficiency and safety of bilateral contemporaneous pallidal stimulation (deep brain stimulation) in levodopa-responsive patients with Parkinson's disease with severe motor fluctuations: a 2-year follow-up review. *Journal of Neurosurgery*, **89**, 713–18.

Gibb, W.R.G., & Lees, A.J. (1987). Clinical and pathological comparisons with postencephalitic parkinsonian syndrome. *Acta Neuropathologica*, **73**, 195–201.

Gnanalingham, K.K., Smith, L.A., Hunter, A.J., Jenner, P., & Marsden, C.D. (1993). Alteration in striatal and extrastriatal D–1 and D–2 dopamine receptors in the MPTP-treated common marmoset: an autoradiographic study. *Synapse*, **14**, 184–94.

Goetz, C.G. (1998). New lessons from old drugs: amantadine and Parkinson's disease. *Neurology*, **50**, 1211–12.

Goetz, C.G., Tanner, C.M., & Glantz, R. (1985). Chronic agonist therapy for Parkinson's disease: a 5-year study of bromocriptine and pergolide. *Neurology*, **35**, 749–51.

Gorell, J.M., Rybicki, B.A., Cole Johnson, C., & Peterson, E.L. (1999). Occupational metal exposures and the risk of Parkinson's disease. *Neuroepidemiology*, **18**, 303–8.

Gowers, W.R. (1896). *A Manual of Disease of the Nervous System*, 2nd edn, pp. 636–57. Philadelphia: Blackston.

Grandy, D.K., Marchionni, M.A., Makan, H., et al. (1989). Cloning of the cDNA and gene for a human D2 dopamine receptor. *Proceedings of the National Academy of Sciences*, **84**, 9762–6.

Gross, R.E., Lombardi, W.J., Lang, A.E., Duff, J., Hutchinson, W.D., & Saint-Cyr, J.A. (1999). Relationship of lesion location to clinical outcome following microelectrode-guided pallidotomy for Parkinson's disease. *Brain*, **122**, 405–16.

Guttman, M. (1997). Double-blind comparison of pramipexole and bromocriptine treatment with placebo in advanced Parkinson's disease. International Pramipexole–Bromocriptine Study Group. *Neurology*, **49**, 1060–5.

Harhangi, B.S., de Rijk, M.C., van Duijin, C.M., Van Broeckhoven, C., Hofman, A., & Breteler, M.M.B. (2000). APOE and the risk of PD with or without dementia in a population-based study. *Neurology*, **54**, 1272–6.

Hartman, D.E., & Abbs, J.H. (1988). Dysarthrias of movement disorders. *Advances in Neurology*, **49**, 289–306.

Haslinger, B., Erhard, P., Kampfe, N., et al. (2001). Event-related functional magnetic resonance imaging in Parkinson's disease before and after levodopa. *Brain*, **124**, 558–70.

Hassler, R., Mundinger, F., & Riechert, T. (1965). Correlations between clinical and autoptic findings in stereotaxic operations of parkinsonism. *Confinia Neurologica*, **26**, 282–90.

Hauser, R.A., Gauger, L., Anderson, W.M., & Zesiewicz, T.A. (2000). Pramipexole-induced somnolence and episodes of daytime sleep. *Movement Disorders*, **15**, 658–63.

Hoehn, M.M., & Yahr, M.D. (1967). Parkinsonism: onset, progression, and mortality. *Neurology*, **17**, 427–42.

Hristova, A.H., & Koller, W.C. (2000). Early Parkinson's disease: what is the best approach to treatment? *Drugs and Aging*, **17**, 165–81.

Hugdahl, K., & Wester, K. (2000). Neurocognitive correlates of stereotactic thalamotomy and thalamic stimulation in parkinsonian patients. *Brain and Cognition*, **42**, 231–52.

Hughes, A.J., Daniel, S.E., Kilford, L., & Lees, A.J. (1992). Accuracy of clinical diagnosis of idiopathic Parkinson's disease: a clinico-pathological study of 100 cases. *Journal of Neurology, Neurosurgery and Psychiatry*, **55**, 181–4.

Hughes, A., Daniel, S., Blankson, S., et al. (1993). A clinicopathologic study of 100 cases of Parkinson's disease. *Archives of Neurology*, **50**,140–8.

Inzelberg, R., Nisipeanu, P., Rabey, J.M., et al. (1996). Double-blind comparison of cabergoline and bromocriptine in Parkinson's disease patients with motor fluctuations. *Neurology*, **47**, 785–8.

Jahanshahi, M., Ardouin, C.M.A., Brown, R.G. et al. (2000). The impact of deep brain stimulation on executive function in Parkinson's disease. *Brain*, **123**, 1142–54.

Jankovic, J. (1987). Pathophysiology and clinical assessment of motor symptoms in Parkinson's Disease. In *Handbook of Parkinson's Disease*, ed. W.C. Koller, pp. 99–126. New York: Raven Press.

Jenkins, A.C. (1966). Epidemiology of parkinsonism in Victoria. *Medical Journal of Australia*, **2**, 496–502.

Kelly, P.J., & Gillingham, F.J. (1980). The long-term results of stereotaxic surgery and L-dopa therapy in patients with Parkinson's disease. A 10-year follow-up study. *Journal of Neurosurgery*, **53**, 332–7.

Koller, W.C., O'Hara, R., Weiner, W.J., et al. (1986). Relationship of aging to Parkinson's Disease. *Advances in Neurology*, **45**, 317–21.

Kostic, V., Przedborski, S., Flaster, E., & Sternic, N. (1991). Early development of levodopa-induced dyskinesias and response fluctuations in young-onset Parkinson's disease. *Neurology*, **41**, 202–5.

Kurlan, R., Richard, I.H., Papka, M., & Marshall, F. (2000). Movement disorders in Alzheimer's disease: more rigidity of definitions is needed. *Movement Disorders*, **15**, 24–9.

Kurland, L.T. (1958). Epidemiology: incidence, geographic distribution and genetic considerations. In *Pathogenesis and Treatment of Parkinsonism*, ed. W.S. Fields, pp. 5–49. Springfield: Charles C. Thomas.

Kurland, L.T., Kurtzke, J.F., Goldberg, I.D., et al. (1987). Parkinsonism. In *Epidemiology of Neurologic and Sense Organ Disorders*, ed. L.F. Kurland, J.F. Kurtzke & I.D. Goldberg, pp. 41–63. Cambridge, MA: Harvard University Press.

Kuzis, G., Sabe, L., Tiberti, C., Dorrego, F., Merello, M., & Starkstein, S.E. (2001). Neuropsychological effects of pallidotomy in patients with parkinson's disease. *Journal of Neurology, Neurosurgery and Psychiatry*, **71**, 563–4.

Lai, E.C., Jankovic, J., Krauss, J.K., Ondo, W.G., & Grossman, R.G. (2000). Long-term efficacy of posteroventral pallidotomy in the treatment of Parkinson's disease. *Neurology*, **55**, 1218–22.

Lang, A.E., Benabid, A.L., Koller, W.C., et al. (1995). The core assessment program for intracerebral transplantation. *Movement Disorders*, **10**, 527–8.

Langston, W.J., & Ballard, P. (1984). Parkinsonism induced by 1-methyl-4-phenyl-1,2,3,6-tetrahydropyridine (MPTP): implications for treatment and the pathogenesis of Parkinson's disease. *Canadian Journal of Neurological Sciences*, **11**, 160–5.

Langtry, H.D., & Clissold, S.P. (1990). Pergolide. A review of its pharmacological properties and therapeutic potential in Parkinson's disease. *Drugs*, **39**, 491–506.

Le Coniat, M., Sokoloff, P., Hillion, J., et al. (1991). Chromosomal localization of the human D–3 dopamine receptor gene. *Human Genetics*, **87**, 618–20.

Lees, A.J., & Stern, G.M. (1981). Sustained bromocriptine therapy in previously untreated patients with Parkinson's disease. *Journal of Neurology, Neurosurgery and Psychiatry*, **44**, 1020–3.

Levy, G. (1966). Kinetics of pharmacologic effects. *Clinical Pharmacology and Therapeutics*, **7**, 362–72.

Lewy, F.H. (1912). Paralysis agitans. I pathologische anatomie. In *Handbuch der Neurologie*, ed. S. Lewandowsky, pp. 920–33. Berlin: Springer.

Lewy, F.H. (1923). *Die Lehre vom Tonus und der Bewegung*. Berlin: Springer.

Lieberman, A.N., Neophytides, A., Leibowitz, M., et al. (1983). Comparative efficacy of pergolide and bromocriptine in patients with advanced Parkinson's disease. *Advances in Neurology*, **37**, 95–108.

Lieberman, A., Ranhosky, A., & Korts, D. (1997). Clinical evaluation of pramipexole in advanced Parkinson's disease: results of a double-blind, placebo-controlled, parallel-group study. *Neurology*, **49**, 162–8.

Limousin, P., Pierre, P.P., Benazzouz, D., Claire, A.A., Hoffmann, D., & Alim-Louis, B. (1998). Electrical stimulation of the subthalamic nucleus in advanced Parkinson's disease. *New England Journal of Medicine*, **339**, 1105–11.

Limousin, P., Pollak, P., & Benazzouz, A., et al. (1995). Bilateral subthalamic nucleus stimulation for severe Parkinson's disease. *Movement Disorders*, **10**, 672–4.

Logemann, J.A. (1988). Dysphagia in movement disorders. Facial dyskinesias. *Advances in Neurology*, **49**, 307–16.

Lombardi, W.J., Gross, R.E., Trepanier, L.L., Lang, A.E., Lozano, A.M., & Saint-Cyr, J.A. (2000). Relationship of lesion location to cognitive outcome following microelectrode-guided pallidotomy for Parkinson's disease. Support for the existence of cognitive circuits in the human pallidum. *Brain*, **123**, 746–58.

Lozano, A.M., Lang, A.E., Galvez-Jimenez, N., et al. (1995). Effect of GPi pallidotomy on motor function in Parkinson's disease. *Lancet*, **346**, 1383–7.

Luginger, E., Wenning, G.K., Bosch, S., & Poewe, W. (2000). Beneficial effects of amantadine on L-dopa induced dyskinesias in Parkinson's disease. *Movement Disorders*, **15**, 873–8.

Masalha, R., Herishanu, Y., Alfahel-Kakunda, A., & Silverman, W.F. (1997). Selective dopamine neurotoxicity by an industrial chemical: an environmental cause of Parkinson's disease? *Brain Research*, 7, 260–4.

McCarter, R.J., Walton, N.H., Rowan, A.F., Gill, S.S., & Palomo, M. (2000). Cognitive functioning after subthalamic nucleotomy for refractory Parkinson's disease. *Journal of Neurology, Neurosurgery and Psychiatry*, 69, 60–6.

McGeer, P.L., McGeer, E.G., & Suzuki, J.S. (1977). Aging and extrapyramidal function. *Archives of Neurology*, 34, 33–5.

Merello, M., & Lees, A.J. (1992). Beginning of dose motor deterioration secondary to L-dopa and apomorphine in Parkinson's disease. *Movement Disorders*, 7, 247.

Merello, M., Hughes, A., Colosimo, C., et al. (1997). Sleep benefit in Parkinson's disease. *Movement Disorders*, 12, 506–8.

Merello, M., Nouzeilles, M.I., Cammarota, A., Betti, O., & Leiguarda, R. (1999a). Comparison of 1-year follow-up evaluations of patients with indication for pallidotomy who did not undergo surgery versus patients with Parkinson's Disease who did undergo pallidotomy: a case control study. *Neurosurgery*, 44, 1–7.

Merello, M., Nouzellies, M.I., Cammarota, A., & Leiguarda, R. (1999b). Effect of memantine (NMDA antagonist) on Parkinson's disease: a double-blind crossover randomized study. *Clinical Neuropharmacology*, 22, 273–6.

Merello, M., Nouzellies, M.I., Kuzis, G., et al. (1999c). Unilateral radiofrequency lesion versus electrostimulation of posteroventral pallidum: a prospective randomized comparison. *Movement Disorders*, 14, 50–6.

Merello, M.J., Lees, A.J., Webster, R., Bovigdon, M., & Gordin, A. (1994). Effect of entacapone, a peripherally acting catechol-O-methyltransferase inhibitor, on the motor response to acute treatment with levodopa in patients with Parkinson's disease. *Journal of Neurology, Neurosurgery and Psychiatry*, 57, 186–9.

Miyawaki, E., Perlmutter, J.S., Tröster, A.I., Videen, T.O., & Koller, W.C. (2000). The behavioral comp44lications of pallidal stimulation: a case report. *Brain and Cognition*, 42, 417–34.

Montastruc, J.L., Chaumerliac, C., Desboeuf, K., et al. (2000). Adverse drug reactions to selegiline: a review of french pharmacovigilance database. *Clinical Neuropharmacology*, 23, 271–5.

Montastruc, J.L., Rascol, O., Senard, J.M., & Rascol, A. (1994). A randomized controlled study comparing bromocriptine to which levodopa was later added, with levodopa alone in previously untreated patients with Parkinson's disease: a five year follow up. *Journal of Neurology, Neurosurgery and Psychiatry*, 1034–8.

Morgante, L., Salemi, G., Meneghini, F., et al. (2000). Parkinson disease survival: a population-based study. *Archives of Neurology*, 57, 507–12.

Morrish, P.K., Rakshi, J.S., Bailey, D.L., Sawle, G.V., & Brooks, D.J. (1998). Measuring the rate of progression and estimating the preclinical period of Parkinson's disease with [18F]dopa PET. *Journal of Neurology, Neurosurgery and Psychiatry*, 64, 314–19.

Nagasaki, Y., Shibazaki, T., Hirai, T., et al. (1986). Long-term follow-up results of selective VIM-thalamotomy. *Journal of Neurosurgery*, **65**, 296–302.

Nutt, J.G., Carter, J.H., Lea, E.S., & Woodward, W.R. (1997a). Motor fluctuations during continuous levodopa infusions in patients with Parkinson's disease. *Movement Disorders*, **12**, 285–92.

Nutt, J.G., Carter, J.H., Van Houten, L., & Woodward, W.R. (1997b). Short- and long-duration responses to levodopa during the first year of levodopa therapy. *Annals of Neurology*, **42**, 349–55.

Nutt, J.G., Gancher, S.T., & Woodward, W.R. (1988). Does an inhibitory action of levodopa contribute to motor fluctuations? *Neurology*, **38**, 1553–7.

Nutt, J.G., Woodward, W.R., Carter, J.H., & Gancher, S.T. (1992). Effect of long-term therapy on the pharmacodynamics of levodopa: relation to on–off phenomenon. *Archives of Neurology*, **49**, 1123–30.

Nutt, J.G., Woodward, W.R., Hammerstad, J.P., et al. (1984). The "On–off" phenomenon in Parkinson's disease: relation to levodopa absorption and transport. *New England Journal of Medicine*, **310**, 483–8.

Ondo, W., Almaguer, M., Jankovic, J., & Simpson, R.K. (2001). Thalamic deep brain stimulation: comparison between unilateral and bilateral placement. *Archives of Neurology*, **58**, 218–22.

Pahwa, R., Wilkinson, S., Smith, D., et al. (1997). High frequency stimulation of the globus pallidus for the treatment of Parkinson's disease. *Neurology*, **49**, 249–53.

Parent, A., & Hazrati, L. (1995). Functional anatomy of the basal ganglia. I. The cortico-basal ganglia-thalamo-cortical loop. *Brain Research Reviews*, **1**, 91–127.

Parkinson, J. (1817). *An Essay on the Shaking Palsy*. London: Sherwood, Neely & Jones.

Parkinson's Disease Research Group in the United Kingdom. (1993). Comparisons of therapeutic effects of levodopa, levodopa and selegiline, and bromocriptine in patients with early, mild Parkinson's disease: three year interim report. *British Medical Journal*, **21**, 469–72.

Parkinson study group (1989). Datatop: a multicenter controlled trial in early Parkinson's disease. *Archives of Neurology*, **46**, 1052–60.

Parkinson study group (1990). Datatop: effect of deprenyl on the progression of disability in early Parkinson's disease. *New England Journal of Medicine*, **322**, 1526–8.

Pillon, B., Ardouin, C., Damier, P., et al. (2000). Neuropsychological changes between "off" and "on" STN or Gpi stimulation in Parkinson's disease. *Neurology*, **55**, 411–18.

Pineda-Trujillo, N., Carvajal-Carmona, L.G., Buritica, O., et al. (2001). A novel Cys212Tyr founder mutation in parkin and allelic heterogeneity of juvenile Parkinsonism in a population from North West Colombia. *Neuroscience Letters*, **298**, 87–90.

Poewe, W. (1993). L-dopa in Parkinson's disease: mechanisms of action and pathophysiology of late failure. In *Parkinson's Disease and Movement Disorders*, ed. J. Jankovic & E. Tolosa, pp. 103–13. Baltimore: William & Wilkins.

Poewe, W., & Granata, R. (1997). Pharmacological treatment of Parkinson's disease. In *Movement Disorders, Neurologic Principles and Practice*, ed. R.L. Watts & W.C. Koller, pp. 201–19. New York: McGraw-Hill.

Poewe, W.H., Lees, A.J., & Stern, G.M. (1986). Low-dose L-DOPA therapy in Parkinson's disease: a 6-year follow-up study. *Neurology*, **36**, 1528–30.

Polymeropoulos, M.H. (2000). Genetics of Parkinson's disease. *Annals of the New York Academy of Sciences*, **920**, 28–32.

Quinn, N. (1999). Progress in functional neurosurgery for Parkinson's disease. *Lancet*, **354**, 1658–9.

Quinn, N., Critchley, P., & Marsden, C.D. (1987). Young onset Parkinson's disease. *Movement Disorders*, **2**, 73–91.

Racette, B.A., McGee-Minnich, L., Moerlein, S.M., Mink, J.W., Videen, T.O., & Perlmutter, J.S. (2001). Welding-related parkinsonism: clinical features, treatment, and pathophysiology. *Neurology*, **56**, 8–13.

Rascol, O., Brooks, D.J., Korczyn, A.D., et al. (2000). A five-year study of the incidence of dyskinesia in patients with early Parkinson's disease who were treated with ropinirole or levodopa. *New England Journal of Medicine*, **342**, 1484–91.

Rascol, O., Sabatini, U., Chollet, F., et al. (1992). Supplementary and primary sensory motor area activity in Parkinson's disease. Regional cerebral blood flow changes during finger movements and effects of apomorphine. *Archives of Neurology*, **49**, 144–8.

Reinmuth, O., Leonard, H.A., Ahlskog, E., Feldman, R., Hershey, L., & Yahr, M.D. (1994). A multicenter double-blind placebo-controlled trial of pergolide as an adjunct of Sinemet in Parkinson's disease. *Movement Disorders*, **9**, 40–7.

Rettig, G.M., York, M.K., Lai, E.C., et al. (2000). Neuropsychological outcome after unilateral pallidotomy for the treatment of Parkinson's disease. *Journal of Neurology, Neurosurgery and Psychiatry*, **69**, 326–36.

Rinne, J.O., Laihinen, A., Nagren, K., et al. (1990). PET demonstrates different behaviour of striatal dopamine D1 and D2 receptors in early Parkinson's disease. *Journal of Neuroscience*, **27**, 494–9.

Rinne, U.K. (1989). Lisuride, a dopamine agonist in the treatment of early Parkinson's disease. *Neurology*, **39**, 336–9.

Rinne, U.K., Bracco, F., Chouza, C., et al. (1997). Cabergoline in the treatment of early Parkinson's disease: results of the first year of treatment in a double-blind comparison of cabergoline and levodopa. The PKDS009 Collaborative Study Group. *Neurology*, **48**, 363–8.

Rubin, A., Lemberger, L., & Dhahir, P. (1981). Physiologic disposition of pergolide. *Journal of Clinical Pharmacology and Therapeutics*, **30**, 258–65.

Sabatini, U., Boulanouar, K., Fabre, N., et al. (2000). Cortical motor reorganization in akinetic patients with Parkinson's disease: a functional MRI study. *Brain*, **123**, 394–403.

Schachter, M., Bedard, P., Debona, A.G., et al., (1980). The role of D-1 and D-2 receptors. *Nature*, **286**, 157–9.

Seibyl, J.P., Marek, K.L., Quinlan, D., et al. (1995). Decreased single-photon emission computed tomographic [123I]beta-CIT striatal uptake correlates with symptom severity in Parkinson's disease. *Annals of Neurology*, **38**, 589–98.

Semchuk, K.M., Love, E.J., & Lee, R.G. (1992). Parkinson's disease and exposure to agricultural work and pesticide chemicals. *Neurology*, **42**, 1328–35.

Sokoloff, P., Giros, B., Martres, M.P., Bouthenet, M.L., & Schwartz, J.C. (1990). Molecular cloning and characterization of a novel dopamine receptor (D3) as a target for neuroleptics. *Nature*, **347**, 146–51.

Spillantini, M.G., & Goedert, M. (2000). The alpha-synucleinopathies: Parkinson's disease, dementia with Lewy bodies, and multiple system atrophy. *Annals of the New York Academy of Sciences*, **920**, 16–27.

Stebbins, G.T., Gabrieli, J.D.E., Shannon, K.M., Penn, R.D., & Goetz, C.G. (2000). Impaired frontostriatal cognitive functioning following posteroventral pallidotomy in advanced Parkinson's disease. *Brain and Cognition*, **42**, 348–63.

Stibe, C.M.H., Lees, A.J., Kempster, P.A., & Stern, G.M. (1988). Subcutaneous apomorphine treatment of parkinsonian on–off fluctuations. *Lancet*, **1**, 232–8.

Sudarsky, L., & Ronthal, M. (1983). Gait disorders among elderly patients. A survey study of 50 patients. *Archives of Neurology*, **40**, 740–3.

Sunahara, R.K., Guan, H.C., O'Dowd, et al. (1991). Cloning of the gene for a human dopamine D5 receptor with higher affinity for dopamine than D1. *Nature*, **350**, 619.

Sweet, R.D., & McDowell, F.H. (1975). Five years' treatment of Parkinson's disease with levodopa: therapeutic results and survival of 100 patients. *Annals of Internal Medicine*, **83**, 456–63.

Tanner, C.M., Chen, B., Wang, W.Z., et al. (1987). Environmental factors in the aetiology of Parkinson's disease. *Canadian Journal of Neurological Sciences*, **14**, 419–23.

Tatsch, K., Schwarz, J., Mozley, P.D., et al. (1997). Relationship between clinical features of Parkinson's disease and presynaptic dopamine transporter binding assessed with [123I]IPT and single-photon emission tomography. *European Journal of Nuclear Medicine*, **24**, 415–21.

Tiberti, M., Jarvie, K.R., Silvia, C., et al. (1991). Cloning, molecular characterization, and chromosomal assignment of a gene encoding a second D1 dopamine receptor subtype: differential expression pattern in rat brain compared with the D-1 receptor. *Proceedings of the National Academy of Sciences*, **87**, 618–20.

Vaamonde, J., Luquin, M.R., & Obeso, J.A. (1991). Subcutaneous lisuride infusion in Parkinson's disease. Response to chronic administration in 34 patients. *Brain*, **114**, 601–14.

Van Tol, H.H.M., Bunzow, J.R., Guan, H.C., et al. (1991). Cloning of the gene for a human dopamine D4 receptor with high affinity for the antipsychotic clozapine. *Nature*, **350**, 610–14.

Verhagen Metman, L., Del Dotto, P., Van den Munckhof, P., Fang, J., Mouradian, M., & Chase, T. (1998). Amantadine as treatment for dyskinesias and motor fluctuations in Parkinson's disease. *Neurology*, **50**, 1323–6.

Weiner, W.J., Nora, L.M., & Gantz, R.H. (1984). Elderly inpatients: postural reflex impairment. *Neurology*, **34**, 945–7.

Werneck, A.L., & Alvarenga, H. (1999). Genetics, drugs and environmental factors in Parkinson's disease. A case-control study. *Arquivos de Neuro-psiquiatria*, **57**, 347–55.

White, W.J., Saint-Cyr, J.A., Tomlinson, R., et al. (1981). Ocular motor deficits in Parkinson's Disease. *Brain*, **2**, 115–29.

Yahr, M.D. (1976). Evaluation of longterm therapy in Parkinson's disease: mortality and therapeutic efficacy. In *Advances in Parkinsonism*, ed. W. Birkmayer & O. Hornykiewicz, pp. 435–43. Basle: Roche.

Yokochi, M., & Narabayashi, H. (1981). Clinical characteristics of juvenile Parkinsonism. In *Research Progress in Parkinson's Disease*, ed. F.C. Rose & R. Capildeo, pp. 35–39. London: Pitman Medical.

Zetusky, W.J., Jankovic, J., & Pirozzolo, F.J. (1985). The heterogeneity of Parkinson's disease: clinical and prognostic implications. *Neurology*, **35**, 522–6.

Chapter 3

Aarsland, D., Litvan, I., & Larsen, J.P. (2001). Neuropsychiatric symptoms of patients with progressive supranuclear palsy and Parkinson's disease. *Journal of Neuropsychiatry and Clinical Neurosciences*, **13**, 42–9.

Adams, R.A., Van Bogaert, L., & Van der Eecken, H. (1964). Striato-nigral degeneration. *Journal of Neuropathology and Experimental Neurology*, **23**, 584–608.

Agid, Y., Javoy-Agid, F., Ruberg, M., et al. (1987). Progressive supranuclear palsy: anatomoclinical and biochemical considerations. *Advances in Neurology*, **45**, 191–206.

Ayd, F.J. (1961). A survey of drug induced extrapyramidal reactions. *Journal of the American Medical Association*, **175**, 1054–60.

Ballard, C., Holmes, C., McKeith, I., et al. (1999). Psychiatric morbidity in dementia with Lewy bodies: a prospective clinical and neuropathological comparative study with Alzheimer's disease. *American Journal of Psychiatry*, **156**, 1039–45.

Ballard, C., McKeith, I., Burn, D., et al. (1997). The UPDRS scale as a means of identifying extrapyramidal signs in patients suffering from dementia with Lewy bodies. *Acta Neurologica Scandinavica*, **96**, 366–71.

Barber, R., Gholkar, A., Scheltens, P., Ballard, C., McKeith, I.G., & O'Brien, J.T. (1999).

Medial temporal lobe atrophy on MRI in dementia with Lewy bodies. *Neurology*, **52**, 1153–8.

Blin, J., Baron, J.C., Dubois, B., et al. (1990). Positron emission tomography study in progressive supranuclear palsy. Brain hypometabolic pattern and clinico-metabolic correlations. *Archives of Neurology*, **47**, 747–52.

Blin, J., Vidailhet, M.J., Pillon, B., Dubois, B., Feve, J.R., & Agid, Y. (1992). Corticobasal degeneration: decreased and asymmetrical glucose consumption as studied with PET. *Movement Disorders*, **7**, 348–54.

Brion, S., Plas, J., & Jeanneau, A. (1991). Maladie de Pick. Point de vue anatomo-clinique. *Revue Neurologique*, **147**, 693–740.

Brooks, D.J. (1994). PET studies in progressive supranuclear palsy. *Journal of Neural Transmission*, **42**, 119–34.

Brooks, D.J. (1996). PET studies in corticobasal degeneration. *Movement Disorders*, **11**, 349.

Bruno, A., & Bruno, S.C. (1966). Effect of L-dopa on pharmacological parkinsonism. *Acta Psychiatrica Scandinavica*, **42**, 264–71.

Brundt, E.R.P., van Weerden, T.W., Pruim, J., & Lakke, J.W.P.F. (1995). Unique myoclonic pattern in corticobasal degeneration. *Movement Disorders*, **10**, 132–42.

Burke, W.J., Pfeiffer, R.F., & McComb, R.D. (1998). Neuroleptic sensitivity to clozapine in dementia with Lewy bodies. *Journal of Neuropsychiatry and Clinical Neurosciences*, **10**, 227–9.

Chen, J.Y., Stern, Y., Sano, M., & Mayeux, R. (1991). Cumulative risks of developing extrapyramidal signs, psychosis, or myoclonus in the course of Alzheimer's disease. *Archives of Neurology*, **48**, 1141–3.

Collins, S.J., Ahlskog, J.E., Parisi, J.E., & Maraganore, D.M. (1995). Progressive supra-nuclear palsy: neuropathologically based diagnostic criteria. *Journal of Neurology, Neurosurgery and Psychiatry*, **58**, 167–73.

Colosimo, C., Albanese, A., Hughes, A.J., de Bruin, V.M., & Lees, A.J. (1995). Some specific clinical features differentiate multiple system atrophy (striatonigral variety) from Parkinson's disease. *Archives of Neurology*, **52**, 294–8.

D'Antona, R., Baron, J.C., Samson, Y., et al. (1985). Subcortical dementia. Frontal cortex hypometabolism detected by positron tomography in patients with progress-ive supranuclear palsy. *Brain*, **108**, 785–99.

Déjèrine, J., & Thomas, A.A. (1900). L'atrophie olivo-ponto-cerebelleuse. *Nouvelle Iconographie du Salpetriere*, **13**, 330–70.

Dickson, D.W., Schmidt, M.L., Lee, V.M., Zhao, M.L., Yen, S.H., & Trojanowski, J.Q. (1994). Immunoreactivity profile of hippocampal CA2/3 neurites in diffuse Lewy body disease. *Acta Neuropathologica*, **87**, 269–76.

Ditter, S.M., & Mirra, S.S. (1987). Neuropathologic and clinical features of Parkinson's disease in Alzheimer's disease patients. *Neurology*, **37**, 754–60.

Fahn, S. (1977). Secondary parkinsonism. In *Scientific Approaches to Clinical Neurology*, ed. E.S. Goldenshohn & S.H. Appel, pp. 1159–89. Philadelphia, PA: Lea & Febiger.

Feany, M.B., Mattiace, L.A., & Dickson, D.W. (1996). Neuropathologic overlap of progressive supranuclear palsy, Pick's disease and corticobasal degeneration. *Journal of Neuropathology and Experimental Neurology*, **55**, 53–67.

Foster, N.L., Gilman, S., Berent, S., Morin, E.M., Brown, M.B., & Koeppe, R.A. (1988). Cerebral hypometabolism in progressive supranuclear palsy studied with positron emission tomography. *Annals of Neurology*, **24**, 399–406.

Friess, E., Kuempfel, T., Winkelmann, J., et al. (2001). Increased growth hormone response to apomorphine in Parkinson disease compared with multiple system atrophy. *Archives of Neurology*, **58**, 241–6.

Funkenstein, H.H., Albert, M.S., Cook, N.R., et al. (1993). Extrapyramidal signs and other neurologic findings in clinically diagnosed Alzheimer's disease. *Archives of Neurology*, 50, 51–6.

Gibb, W.R.G., Luthert, P.J., & Marsden, C.D. (1989). Corticobasal degeneration. *Brain*, **112**, 1171–92.

Gibb, W.R.C., Luthert, P.J., & Marsden, C.D. (1991). Clinical and pathological features of corticobasal degeneration. *Advances in Neurology*, **53**, 51–4.

Gilman, S., Low, P.A., Quinn, N., et al. (1999). Consensus statement on the diagnosis of multiple system atrophy. *Journal of Neurological Sciences*, **163**, 94–8.

Golbe, L.I. (1992). Epidemiology. In *Progressive Supranuclear Palsy: Clinical and Research Approaches*, ed. I. Litvan & Y. Agid, pp. 33–43. New York: Oxford University Press.

Golbe, L.I., Davis, P.H., Schoenberg, B.S., & Duvoisin, R.C. (1988). Prevalence and natural history of progressive supranuclear palsy. *Neurology*, **38**, 1031–4.

Grisoli, M., Fetoni, V., Savoiardo, M., Girotti, F., & Bruzzone, M.G. (1995). MRI in corticobasal degeneration. *European Journal of Neurology*, **2**, 547–52.

Hauser, R.A., Murtaugh, F.R., & Olanow, C.W. (1996). Magnetic resonance imaging (MRI) in corticobasal degeneration. *Movement Disorders*, **11**, 352.

Hauw, J.J., Daniel, S.E., Dickson, D., et al. (1994). Preliminary NINDS neuropathologic criteria for Steele–Richardson–Olszewski syndrome (progressive supranuclear palsy). *Neurology*, **44**, 2015–19.

Holmes, C., Cairns, N., Lantos, P., & Mann, A. (1999). Validity of current clinical criteria for Alzheimer's disease, vascular dementia and dementia with Lewy bodies. *British Journal of Psychiatry*, **174**, 45–50.

Hu, X.S., Okamura, N., Arai, H., et al. (2000). ^{18}F-fluorodopa PET study of striatal dopamine uptake in the diagnosis of dementia with Lewy bodies. *Neurology*, **55**, 1575–6.

Hughes, A.J., Ben-Shlomo, Y., Daniel, S.E., & Lees, A.J. (1992a). What features improve the accuracy of clinical diagnosis in Parkinson's disease? *Neurology*, **42**, 1142–6.

Hughes, A.J., Daniel, S.E., Kilford, L., & Lees, A.J. (1992b). Accuracy of clinical diagnosis of idiopathic Parkinson's disease: a clinico-pathological study of 100 cases. *Journal of Neurology, Neurosurgery and Psychiatry*, **55**, 181–4.

Ikeda, K., Kotabe, T., Kanbashi, S., & Kinoshita, M. (1996). Parkinsonism in lacunar infarcts of the basal ganglia. *European Neurology*, **36**, 248–9.

Ishii, K., Yamaji, S., Kitagaki, H., Imamura, T., Hirono, N., & Mori, E. (1999). Regional cerebral blood flow difference between dementia with Lewy bodies and AD. *Neurology*, **53**, 413–16.

Konagaya, M., Konagaya, Y., & Lida, M. (1994). Clinical and magnetic resonance imaging study of extrapyramidal symptoms in multiple system atrophy. *Journal of Neurology, Neurosurgery and Psychiatry*, **57**, 1528–31.

Kosaka, K., Yoshimura, M., Ikeda, K., et al. (1984). Diffuse type of Lewy body disease: progressive dementia with abundant cortical Lewy bodies and senile changes of various degree – a new disease? *Clinical Neuropathology*, **3**, 185–92.

Kraepelin, E. (1921). *Lectures on Clinical Psychiatry*. New York: Hafner.

Lang, A.E. (1992). Cortical basal ganglionic degeneration presenting with "progressive loss of speech output and orofacial dyspraxia". *Journal of Neurology, Neurosurgery and Psychiatry*, **55**, 1101.

Langlais, P.J., Thal, L., Hansen, L., Galasko, D., Alford, M., & Masliah, E. (1993). Neurotransmitters in basal ganglia and cortex of Alzheimer's disease with and without Lewy bodies. *Neurology*, **43**, 1927–34.

Lantos, P.L. (1995). Neuropathological diagnostic criteria of multiple system atrophy: a review. In *Neuropathological Diagnostic Criteria for Brain Banking*, ed. F.F. Cruz-Sanchez, R. Ravid & M.L. Cuzner, pp. 116–21. Amsterdam: IOS Press.

Leenders, K.L., Frackowiak, R.S., & Lees, A.J. (1988). Steele–Richardson–Olszewski syndrome. Brain energy metabolism, blood flow and fluorodopa uptake measured by positron emission tomography. *Brain*, **111**, 615–30.

Leiguarda, R.C., Lees, A.J., Merello, M., Starkstein, S., & Marsden, C.D. (1994). The nature of apraxia in corticobasal degeneration. *Journal of Neurology, Neurosurgery and Psychiatry*, **57**, 455–9.

Litvan, I., Agid, Y., Calne, D., et al. (1996). Clinical research criteria for the diagnosis of progressive supranuclear palsy (Steele–Richardson–Olszewski syndrome): report of the NINDS-SPSP international workshop. *Neurology*, **47**, 1–9.

Litvan, I., Agid, Y., Goetz, C., et al. (1997). Accuracy of the clinical diagnosis of corticobasal degeneration: a clinicopathologic study. *Neurology*, **48**, 119–25.

Louis, E.D., Klatka, L.A., Liu, Y., & Fahn, S. (1997). Comparison of extrapyramidal features in 31 pathologically confirmed cases of diffuse Lewy body disease and 34 pathologically confirmed cases of Parkinson's disease. *Neurology*, **48**, 376–80.

Magalhaes, M., Wenning, G.K., Daniel, S.E., & Quinn, N.P. (1995). Autonomic dysfunction in pathologically confirmed multiple system atrophy and idiopathic

Parkinson's disease – a retrospective comparison. *Acta Neurologica Scandinavica*, **91**, 98–102.

Marti Masso, J.F., Carrera, N., & Urtasun, M. (1991). Drugs inducing Parkinsonism in our environment. *Journal of Neurology, Neurosurgery and Psychiatry*, **54**, 1025.

McKeith, I.G., Ballard, C.G., Perry, R.H., et al. (2000). Prospective validation of consensus criteria for the diagnosis of dementia with Lewy bodies. *Neurology*, **54**, 1050–8.

McKeith, I.G., Galasko, D., Kosaka, K., et al. (1996). Consensus guidelines for the clinical and pathological diagnosis of dementia with Lewy bodies (DLB): report of the consortium on DLB International Workshop. *Neurology*, **47**, 911–22.

McKeith, I.G., Perry, R.H., Fairbairn, A.F., Jabeen, S., & Perry, E.K. (1992). Operational criteria for senile dementia of Lewy body type (SDLT). *Psychological Medicine*, **22**, 911–22.

McLolland, H.A. (1978). Discussion on assessment of drug-induced extrapyramidal reactions. *British Journal of Psychiatry*, **132**, 27–30.

Mega, M.S., Masterman, D.L., Benson, D.F., et al. (1996). Dementia with Lewy bodies: reliability and validity of clinical and pathologic criteria. *Neurology*, **47**, 1403–9.

Merello, M., Sabe, L., Teson, A., et al. (1994). Extrapyramidalism in Alzheimer's disease: prevalence, psychiatric, and neuropsychological correlates. *Journal of Neurology, Neurosurgery and Psychiatry*, **57**, 1503–9.

Merello, M., Starkstein, S., Petracca, G., Amado Cataneo, E., Manes, F., & Leiguarda, R. (1996). Drug induced parkinsonism in schizophrenic patients: motor response and psychiatric changes after acute challenge with L-dopa and apomorphine. *Clinical Neuropharmacology*, **19**, 439–43.

Mindham, R.H.S. (1976). Assessment of drug-induced extrapyramidal reactions and of drugs given for their control. *British Journal of Clinical Pharmacology*, **3** (Suppl. 2), 395–400.

Molsa, P.K., Marttila, R.J., & Rinne, U.K. (1984). Extrapyramidal signs in Alzheimer's disease. *Neurology*, **34**, 1114–16.

Muller, J., Wenning, G.K., Verny, M., et al. (2001). Progression of dysarthria and dysphagia in postmortem-confirmed parkinsonian disorders. *Archives of Neurology*, **58**, 259–64.

Olanow, C.W. (1992). Magnetic resonance imaging in parkinsonism. *Neurologic Clinics*, **10**, 405–20.

Olichney, J.M., Galasko, D., Salmon, D.P., et al. (1998). Cognitive decline is faster in Lewy body variant than in Alzheimer's disease. *Neurology*, **51**, 351–7.

Owens, D.G.C., Johnstone, E.C., & Frith, C.D. (1982). Spontaneous involuntary disorders of movements, their prevalence, severity and distribution in chronic schizophrenia with and without treatment with neuroleptics. *Archives of General Psychiatry*, **39**, 452–61.

Papp, M.I., & Lantos, P.L. (1992). Accumulation of tubular structures in oligodendroglial and neuronal cells as the basic alteration in multiple system atrophy. *Journal of Neurological Sciences*, **107**, 172–82.

Perry, R., McKeith, I., & Perry, E. (1997). Lewy body dementia – clinical, pathological and neurochemical interconnections. *Journal of Neural Transmission*, **51**, 95–109.

Perry, R.H., Irving, D., Blessed, G., Fairbairn, A., & Perry, E.K. (1990). Senile dementia of the Lewy body type: a clinically and neuropathologically distinct form of Lewy body dementia in the elderly. *Journal of Neurological Sciences*, **95**, 119–39.

Piggott, M.A., Marshall, E.F., Thomas, N., et al. (1999). Striatal dopaminergic markers in dementia with Lewy bodies, Alzheimer's and Parkinson's diseases: rostrocaudal distribution. *Brain*, **122**, 1449–68.

Pillon, B., Vidailhet, M., Sirigu, A., Agid, Y., & Dubois, B. (1996). The cognitive syndrome of corticobasal degeneration. *Movement Disorders*, **11**, 354.

Quinn, N. (1995). Parkinsonism-recognition and differential diagnosis. *British Medical Journal*, **310**, 447–52.

Rajput, A.H., Rozdilsky, B., & Rajput, A. (1991). Accuracy of clinical diagnosis in parkinsonism: a prospective study. *Canadian Journal of Neurological Sciences*, **18**, 275–8.

Rebeiz, J.J., Kolodny, E.H., & Richardson, E.P. (1968). Corticodentatonigral degeneration with neuronal achromasia. *Archives of Neurology*, **18**, 20–33.

Reider-Grosswasser, I., Bornstein, N.M., & Korczyn, A.D. (1995). Parkinsonism in patients with lacunar infarcts of the basal ganglia. *European Neurology*, **35**, 46–9.

Revesz, T., Geddes, J.F., & Daniel, S.E. (1995). Corticobasal degeneration. In *Neuropathological Diagnostic Criteria for Brain Banking*, ed. F.F. Cruz-Sanchez, R. Ravid & M.L. Cuzner, pp. 99–104. Amsterdam: IOS Press.

Riley, D.E., Lang, A.E., Lewis, A., et al. (1990). Cortical-basal ganglionic degeneration. *Neurology*, **40**, 1203–12.

Savoiardo, M., Girotti, F., Strada, L., & Ciceri, E. (1994). Magnetic resonance imaging in progressive supranuclear palsy and other parkinsonian disorders. *Journal of Neural Transmission*, **42**, 93–110.

Sawle, G.V., Brooks, D.J., Marsden, C.D., & Frackowiak, R.S. (1991). Corticobasal degeneration. A unique pattern of regional cortical oxygen hypometabolism and striatal fluorodopa uptake demonstrated by positron emission tomography. *Brain*, **114**, 541–56.

Schultz, J.B., Klockgether, T., & Petersen, D. (1999). Multiple system atrophy: natural history, MRI morphology, and dopamine receptor imaging with [123]IBZM-SPECT. *Journal of Neurology, Neurosurgery and Psychiatry*, **57**, 1047–56.

Shy, G.M., & Drager, G.A. (1960). A neurologic syndrome associated with orthostatic hypotension. *Archives of Neurology*, **2**, 511–27.

Soliveri P., Monza D., Paridi D., et al. (2000). Neuropsychological follow up in patients with Parkinson's disease, striatonigral degeneration-type multisystem atrophy, and progressive supranuclear palsy. *Journal of Neurology, Neurosurgery and Psychiatry*, **69**, 313–18.

Starkstein, S.E., Petracca, G., Chemerinski, E., & Merello, M. (2001). Prevalence and correlates of Parkinsonism in patients with primary depression. *Neurology* (in press).

Starkstein, S.E., Petracca, G., Teson, A., et al. (1996). Catatonia in depression: prevalence, clinical correlates, and validation of a scale. *Journal of Neurology, Neurosurgery and Psychiatry*, **60**, 326–32.

Steele, J.C., Richardson, J.C., & Olszewski, J. (1964). Progressive supranuclear palsy. *Archives of Neurology*, **10**, 333–59.

Talbot, P.R., Lloyd, J.J., Snowden, J.S., Neary, D., & Testa, H.J. (1998). A clinical role for ^{99m}Tc-HMPAO SPECT in the investigation of dementia? *Journal of Neurology, Neurosurgery and Psychiatry*, **64**, 306–13.

Tolosa, E.S., & Santamaria, J. (1984). Parkinsonism and basal ganglia infarcts. *Neurology*, **34**, 1516–18.

van Royen, E., Verhoeff, N.F., Speelman, J.D., Wolters, E.C., Kuiper, M.A., & Janssen, A.G. (1993). Multiple system atrophy and progressive supranuclear palsy. Diminished striatal D2 dopamine receptor activity demonstrated by 123-IBZM single photon emission computed tomography. *Archives of Neurology*, **50**, 513–16.

Verny, M., Duyckaerts, C., Agid, Y., & Hauw, J.J. (1996). The significance of cortical pathology in progressive supranuclear palsy: clinicopathological data in 10 cases. *Brain*, **119**, 1123–36.

Walker, M.P., Ayre, G.A., Cummings, J.L., et al. (2000). The clinician assessment of fluctuation and the one day fluctuation assessment scale. Two methods to assess fluctuating confusion in dementia. *British Journal of Psychiatry*, **177**, 252–6.

Wenning, G.K., Ben-Shlomo, Y., Magalhaes, M., Daniel, S.E., & Quinn, N.P. (1995). Clinicopathological study of 35 cases of multiple system atrophy. *Journal of Neurology, Neurosurgery and Psychiatry*, **58**, 160–6.

Winikates, J., & Jankovic, J. (1999). Clinical correlates of vascular parkinsonism. *Archives of Neurology*, **56**, 98–102.

Zijlmans, J.C.M., Thijssen, H.O.M., Vogels, O.J.M., et al. (1995). MRI in patients suspected of vascular parkinsonism. *Neurology*, **45**, 2183–8.

Chapter 4

Ackermann, H., & Ziegler, W. (1996). Articulatory deficits in Parkinsonian dysarthria: an acoustic analysis. *Journal of Neurology, Neurosurgery and Psychiatry*, **54**, 1093–8.

Agid, Y., Graybiel, A.M., & Ruberg, M. (1990). The efficacy of levodopa treatment declines in the course of Parkinson's disease. Do not dopaminergic lesions play a role? *Advances in Neurology*, **53**, 83–100.

Agid, Y., Javoy-Agid, F., & Ruberg, M. (1987). Biochemistry of neurotransmitters in Parkinson's disease. In *Movement Disorders. 2. Neurology*, Vol. 7, ed. C.D. Marsden & S. Fahn, pp. 166–230. London: Butterworths.

Agostino, R., Hallett, M., & Sanes, J.N. (1996). Motor skill learning in Parkinson's disease. *Journal of Neurological Sciences*, **139**, 218–26.

Alexander, G.E., De Long, M.R., & Strick, P.L. (1986). Parallel organization of functionally segregated circuits linking basal ganglia and cortex. *Annual Review of Neurosciences*, **9**, 357–81.

American Psychiatric Association (1994). *Diagnostic and Statistical Manual of Mental Disorders – DSM-IV*. Washington, DC: American Psychiatric Press.

Arendt, T., Bigl, V., Arendt, A., & Tennstedt, A. (1983). Loss of neurons in the nucleus basalis of Meynert in Alzheimer's disease. *Acta Neuropathologica*, **61**, 101–8.

Asahina, M., Suhara, T., Shinotoh, H., Inove, O., Suzuki, K., & Hattori, T. (1998). Brain muscarinic receptors in progressive supranuclear palsy and Parkinson's disease: a positron emission tomographic study. *Journal of Neurology, Neurosurgery and Psychiatry*, **65**, 155–63.

Bayles, K.A., Tomoeda, C.K., Wood, J.A., et al. (1996). Change in cognitive function in idiopathic Parkinson disease. *Archives of Neurology*, **53**, 1140–6.

Bédard, M.A., El Massioui, F., Malapani, C., et al. (1998). Attentional deficits in Parkinson's disease: partial reversibility with naphtoxazine (SDZ NVI-085), a selective noradrenergic α1 agonist. *Clinical Neuropharmacology*, **21**, 108–17.

Bédard, M.A., Pillon, B., Dubois, B., Duchesne, N., Masson, H., & Agid, Y. (1999). Acute and long-term administration of anticholinergics in Parkinson's disease: specific effects on the subcortico-frontal syndrome. *Brain and Cognition*, **40**, 289–313.

Benke, T.H., Hohenstein, C., Poewe, W., & Butterworth, B. (2000). Repetitive speech phenomena in Parkinson's disease. *Journal of Neurology, Neurosurgery and Psychiatry*, **69**, 319–25.

Benton, A.L. (1968). Differential behavioral effects in frontal lobe disease. *Neuropsychologia*, **6**, 53–60.

Berger, H.J.C., van Es, N., van Spaendonck, K.P.M., et al. (1999). Relationship between memory strategies and motor symptoms in Parkinson's disease. *Journal of Clinical and Experimental Neuropsychology*, **21**, 677–84.

Biggins, C.A., Boyd, J.L., & Harrop, F.M. (1992). A controlled longitudinal study of dementia in Parkinson's disease. *Journal of Neurology, Neurosurgery and Psychiatry*, **55**, 566–71.

Blonder, L.X., Gur, R.E., & Gur, R.C. (1989). The effects of right and left hemiparkinsonism on prosody. *Brain and Language*, **36**, 193–207.

Boller, F., Mizutani, T., Roessmann, U., & Gambetti, P. (1980). Parkinson disease, dementia, and Alzheimer disease: clinicopathological correlations. *Annals of Neurology*, **7**, 329–35.

Bondi, N.W., & Kazniak, A.W. (1991). Implicit and explicit memory in Alzheimer's disease and Parkinson's disease. *Journal of Clinical and Experimental Neuropsychology*, **13**, 339–58.

Borod, J.C., Welkowitz, J.M.A., Brozgold, A.Z., Martin, C., Peselow, E., & Diller, L. (1990). Parameters of emotional processing in neuropsychiatric disorders: conceptual issues and a battery of tests. *Journal of Communication Disorders*, **23**, 247–71.

Braak, H., de Vos, R.A.I., Jansen, E.N.H., Bratzke, H., & Braak, E. (1998). Neuropathological hallmarks of Alzheimer's and Parkinson's diseases. *Progress in Brain Research*, **117**, 267–85.

Brown, R.G., & Marsden, C.D. (1984). How common is dementia in Parkinson's disease? *Lancet*, **2**, 1262–5.

Brown, R.G., & Marsden, C.D. (1990). Cognitive function in Parkinson's disease: from description to theory. *Trends in Neurosciences*, **13**, 21–9.

Burkhardt, C.R., Filley, C.M., Kleinschmidt-DeMasters, B.K., de la Monte, S., Norenberg, M.D., & Schneck, S.A. (1988). Diffuse Lewy body disease and progressive dementia. *Neurology*, **38**, 1520–8.

Buytenhuijs, E.L., Berger, H.J.C., Van Spaendonck, K.P.M., Horstink, M.W.I.M., Born, G.F., & Cools, A.R. (1994). Memory and learning strategies in patients with Parkinson's disease. *Neuropsychologia*, **32**, 335–42.

Caekebeke, J.F.V., Jennekens-Schinkel, A., van der Linden, M.E., Buruma, O.J.S., & Ross, R.A.C. (1991). The interpretation of dysprosody in patients with Parkinson's disease. *Journal of Neurology, Neurosurgery and Psychiatry*, **54**, 145–8.

Canavan, A.G.M., Passingham, R.E., & Marsden, C.D. (1990). Prism adaptation and other tasks involving spatial abilities in patients with Parkinson's disease, patients with frontal lobe lesions and patients with unilateral temporal lobectomies. *Neuropsychologia*, **28**, 969–84.

Candy, J.M., Perry, R.H., & Perry, E.K. (1983). Pathological changes in the nucleus of Meynert in Alzheimer's disease. *Journal of Neurological Sciences*, **54**, 277–89.

Caparros-Lefebvre, D., Pécheux, N., Petit, V., Duhamel, A., & Petit, H. (1995). Which factors predict cognitive decline in Parkinson's disease? *Journal of Neurology, Neurosurgery and Psychiatry*, **58**, 51–5.

Cash, R., Dennis, T., L'Heureux, R., Raisman, R., Javoy-Agid, F., & Scatton, B. (1987). Parkinson's disease and dementia: norepinephrine and dopamine in locus ceruleus. *Neurology*, **37**, 42–6.

Charcot, J.M. (1875, 1985). *Leçons sur les Maladies du Système Nerveux*, 2nd edn, p. 179. Paris: Delahaye.

Chui, H.C., Lyness, S.A., Sobel, E., & Scheneider, L.S. (1994). Extrapyramidal signs and psychiatric symptoms predict faster cognitive decline in Alzheimer's disease. *Archives of Neurology*, **51**, 676–81.

Churchyard, A., & Lees, A.J. (1997). The relationship between dementia and direct involvement of the hippocampus and amygdala in Parkinson's disease. *Neurology*, **49**, 1570–6.

Cooper, J.A., Sagar, H.J., & Jordan, N. (1991). Cognitive impairment in early untreated Parkinson's disease and its relationship to motor disability. *Brain*, **114**, 2095–122.

Cooper, J.A., Sagar, H.J., & Sullivan, E.V. (1993). Short-term memory and temporal ordering in early Parkinson's disease: effects of disease chronicity and medication. *Neuropsychologia*, **31**, 933–49.

Cooper, J.A., Sagar, H.J., Tidswell, P., & Jordan, N. (1994). Slowed central processing in simple and go/no-go reaction time tasks in Parkinson's disease. *Brain*, **117**, 517–29.

Crucian, G.P., Barrett, A.M., Schwartz, R.L., et al. (1999). Cognitive and vestibulo-proprioceptive components of spatial ability in Parkinson's disease. *Neuropsychologia*, **38**, 757–67.

Cummings, J.L. (1993). Frontal-subcortical circuits and human behavior. *Archives of Neurology*, **50**, 873–80.

Cummings, J.L., & Benson, D.F. (1984). Subcortical dementia. Review of an emerging concept. *Archives of Neurology*, **41**, 874–9.

Cummings, J.L., Darkins, A., Mendez, M., Hill, M.A., & Benson, D.F. (1988). Alzheimer's disease and Parkinson's disease: comparison of speech and language alterations. *Neurology*, **38**, 680–4.

Dalrymple-Alford, J.C., Kalders, A.S., Jones, R.D., & Watson, R.W. (1994). A central executive deficit in patients with Parkinson's disease. *Journal of Neurology, Neurosurgery and Psychiatry*, **57**, 360–7.

Darkins, A.W., Fromkin, V.A., & Benson, D.F. (1988). A characterization of the prosodic loss in Parkinson's disease. *Brain and Language*, **34**, 315–27.

Davidson, O.R., & Knight, R.G. (1995). Speed of semantic reasoning and mental rotation in patients with Parkinson's disease without dementia. *Neuropsychiatry, Neuropsychology, and Behavioral Neurology*, **8**, 182–8.

de la Monte, S.M., Wells, S.E., Hedley-Whyte, E.T., & Growdon, J.H. (1989). Neuropathological distinction between Parkinson's dementia and Parkinson's plus Alzheimer's disease. *Annals of Neurology*, **26**, 309–20.

Dubois, B., & Pillon, B. (1997). Cognitive deficits in Parkinson's disease. *Journal of Neurology*, **244**, 2–8.

Dubois, B., Boller, F., Pillon, B., & Agid, Y. (1991). Cognitive deficits in Parkinson's disease. In *Handbook of Neuropsychology*, ed. F. Boller & J. Grafman, Vol. 5, pp. 195–240. Amsterdam: Elsevier.

Dujardin, K., Duhamel, A., Becquet, E., Grunberg, C., Defebvre, L., & Destee, A. (1999). Neuropsychological abnormalities in first degree relatives of patients with familial Parkinson's disease. *Journal of Neurology, Neurosurgery and Psychiatry*, **67**, 323–8.

Duncombe, M.E., Bradshaw, J.L., Iansek, R., & Phillips, J.G. (1994). Parkinsonian patients without dementia or depression do not suffer from bradyphrenia as indexed by performance in mental rotation tasks with and without advanced information. *Neuropsychologia*, **32**, 1383–96.

Duret, M., Goldman, D., Messina, J., & Hildebrand, J. (1989). Effect of L-dopa on dementia related rigidity. *Acta Neurologica Scandinavica*, **80**, 64–7.

Ebmeier, K.P., Calder, S.A., & Crawford, J.R. (1990). Clinical features predicting dementia in idiopathic Parkinson's disease: a follow up study. *Neurology*, **40**, 1222–4.

Ellis, R.J., Caligiuri, M., Galasko, D., & Thal, L. (1996). Extrapyramidal motor signs in clinically diagnosed Alzheimer's disease. *Alzheimer Disease and Associated Disorders*, **10**, 103–14.

Erkinjuntti, T., Ostbye, T., Steenhuis, R., & Hachinski, V. (1997). The effect of different diagnostic criteria on the prevalence of dementia. *New England Journal of Medicine*, **377**, 1667–74.

Fahn, S., & Elton, R.I. (1987). UPDRS Development Committee: Unified Parkinson's Disease Rating Scale. *Recent Developments in Parkinson's Disease*, ed. S. Fahn, C.D. Marsden, D. Calne & M. Golstein, pp. 153–63. Florham Park, NJ: Macmillan Healthcare Information.

Funkenstein, H.H., Albert, M.S., & Cook, N.R. (1993). Extrapyramidal signs and other neuroleptic findings in clinically diagnosed Alzheimer's disease. *Archives of Neurology*, **50**, 51–6.

Glatt, S.L., Hubble, J.P., Lyons, K., et al. (1996). Risk factors for dementia in Parkinson's disease: effect of education. *Neuroepidemiology*, **15**, 20–5.

Goldman, W.P., Baty, J.D., Buckles, V.D., Sahrmann, S., & Morris, J.C. (1998). Cognitive and motor functioning in Parkinson disease. *Archives of Neurology*, **55**, 674–80.

Graham, J.M., & Sagar, H.J. (1999). A data-driven approach to the study of heterogeneity in idiopathic Parkinson's disease: identification of three distinct subtypes. *Movement Disorders*, **14**, 10–20.

Growdon, J.H., Corkin, S., & Rosen, T.J. (1990). Distinctive aspects of cognitive dysfunction in Parkinson's disease. *Advances in Neurology*, **53**, 365–76.

Haaland, K.Y., Harrington, D.L., O'Brien, S., & Hermanowicz, N. (1997). Cognitive-motor learning in Parkinson's disease. *Neuropsychology*, **11**, 180–6.

Haroutunian, V., Serby, M., Purohit, D.P. et al. (2000). Contribution of Lewy body inclusions to dementia in patients with and without Alzheimer disease neuropsychological conditions. *Archives of Neurology*, **57**, 1145–50.

Hayashi, R., Hanyu, N., Kurashima, T., Tokutake, T., & Yanagisawa, N. (1996). Relationship between cognitive impairment, event-related potentials, and motor disability scores in patients with Parkinson's disease: 2-year follow-up study. *Journal of Neurological Sciences*, **141**, 45–8.

Heikkilä, V.M., Turkka, J., Korpelainen, J., Kallanranta, T., & Summala, H. (1998). Decreased driving ability in people with Parkinson's disease. *Journal of Neurology, Neurosurgery and Psychiatry*, **64**, 325–30.

Heindel, W.C., Salmon, D.P., Shults, C.W., Walicke, P.A., Butters, N. (1989). Neuropsychological evidence for multiple implicit memory systems: a comparison of Alzheimer's, Huntington's, and Parkinson's disease patients. *Journal of Neuroscience*, **9**, 582–7.

Helscher, R.J., & Pinter, M.M. (1993). Speed and power of higher cerebral functions in parkinsonian patients. *Journal of Neural Transmission*, **5**, 35–44.

Ho, A.K., Iansek, R., & Bradshaw, J.L. (1999). Regulation of parkinsonian speech volume: the effect of interlocutor distance. *Journal of Neurology, Neurosurgery and Psychiatry*, **67**, 199–202.

Hobson, P., & Meara, J. (1999). The detection of dementia and cognitive impairment in a community population of elderly people with Parkinson's disease by use of the CAMCOG neuropsychological test. *Age and Ageing*, **28**, 39–43.

Hodgson, T.L., Dittrich, W.H., Henderson, L., & Kennard, C. (1999). Eye movements and spatial working memory in Parkinson's disease. *Neuropsychologia*, **37**, 927–38.

Holthoff-Detto, V.A., Kessler, J., Herholz, K., et al. (1997). Functional effects of striatal dysfunction in Parkinson's disease. *Archives of Neurology*, **54**, 145–50.

Hu, M.T., Taylor-Robinson, S.D., Chaudhuri, K.R., et al. (1999). Evidence for cortical dysfunction in clinically non-demented patients with Parkinson's disease: a proton MR spectroscopy study. *Journal of Neurology, Neurosurgery and Psychiatry*, **67**, 20–6.

Hu, M.T.M., Taylor-Robinson, S.D., Chaudhuri, K.R., et al. (2000). Cortical dysfunction in non-demented Parkinson's disease patients. A combined ^{31}P-MRS and ^{18}FDG-PET study. *Brain*, **123**, 340–52.

Hughes, A.J., Daniel, S.E., Blankson, S., & Lees, A.J. (1993). A clinicopathologic study of 100 cases of Parkinson's disease. *Archives of Neurology*, **50**, 140–8.

Hughes, T.A., Ross, H.F., Musa, S., et al. (2000). A 10-year study of the incidence of and factors predicting dementia in Parkinson's disease. *Neurology*, **54**, 1596–603.

Hurtig, H.I., Trojanowski, J.Q., Galvin, J., et al. (2000). Alpha-synuclein cortical Lewy bodies correlate with dementia in Parkinson's disease. *Neurology*, **54**, 1916–21.

Illes, J. (1989). Neurolinguistic features of spontaneous language production dissociate three forms of neurodegenerative disease. *Brain and Language*, **37**, 628–42.

Ince, P., Irving, D., MacArthur, F., & Perry, R.H. (1991). Quantified neuropathological study of Alzheimer-type pathology in the hippocampus: comparison of senile dementia of Alzheimer type, senile dementia of Lewy body type, Parkinson's disease and non-demented elderly control patients. *Journal of the Neurological Sciences*, **106**, 142–52.

Ivory, S.J., Knight, R.G., Longmore, B.E., & Caradoc-Davies, T. (1999). Verbal memory in non-demented patients with idiopathic Parkinson's disease. *Neuropsychologia*, **37**, 817–28.

Jankovic, J., McDermott, M., & Carter, J. (1990). Variable expression of Parkinson's disease. A base-line analysis of the DATATOP cohort. *Neurology*, **40**, 1529–34.

Jendroska, K. (1997). The relationship of Alzheimer-type pathology to dementia in Parkinson's disease. *Journal of Neural Transmission*, **49**, 23–31.

Katzen, H.L., Levin, B.E., & Llabre, M.L. (1998). Age of disease onset influences cognition in Parkinson's disease. *Journal of International Neuropsychological Society*, **4**, 285–90.

Kazee, A.M., Cox, C., & Richfield, E.K. (1995). Substantia nigra lesions in Alzheimer disease and normal aging. *Alzheimer Disease and Associated Disorders*, **9**, 61–7.

Koening, O., Thomas-Antérion, C., & Laurent, B. (1999). Procedural learning in Parkinson's disease: intact and impaired cognitive components. *Neuropsychologia*, **37**, 1103–9.

Kuzis, G., Sabe, L., Tiberti, C., Merello, M., Leiguarda, R., & Starkstein, S.E. (1999). Explicit and implicit learning in patients with Alzheimer disease and Parkinson disease with dementia. *Neuropsychiatry, Neuropsychology, and Behavioral Neurology*, **12**, 265–9.

Laasko, M.P., Partanen, K., Riekkinen, P., et al. (1996). Hippocampal volumes in Alzheimer disease, Parkinson's disease with and without dementia, and in vascular dementia: an MRI study. *Neurology*, **46**, 678–81.

Langlais, P.J., Thal, L., Hansen, L., Galasko, D., Alford, M., & Masliah, E. (1993). Neurotransmitters in basal ganglia and cortex of Alzheimer's disease with and without Lewy bodies. Neurology, 43, 1927–34.

Lees, A.J., & Smith, E. (1983). Cognitive deficits in the early stages of Parkinson's disease. *Brain*, **106**, 257–70.

Leplow, B., Dierks, Ch., Herrmann, P., Pieper, N., Annecke, R., & Ulm, G. (1997). Remote memory in Parkinson's disease and senile dementia. *Neuropsychologia*, **35**, 547–57.

Levin, B.E., & Katzen, H.L. (1995). Early cognitive changes and nondementing behavioral abnormalities in Parkinson's disease. *Advances in Neurology*, **65**, 85–95.

Levin, B.E., Llabre, B.M., & Weiner, W.J. (1989). Cognitive impairments associated with early Parkinson's disease. *Neurology*, **39**, 557–61.

Levin, B.E., Llabre, M.M., Reisman, S., et al. (1991). Visuospatial impairment in Parkinson's disease. *Neurology*, **41**, 365–9.

Lewis, F.M., Lapointe, L., Murdoch, B.E., & Chenery, H.J. (1998). Language impairment in Parkinson's disease. *Aphasiology*, **12**, 193–206.

Litvan, Y., Mohr, E., Williams, J., Gomez, C., & Chase, T.N. (1991). Differential memory and executive functions in demented patients with Parkinson's and Alzheimer's disease. *Journal of Neurology, Neurosurgery and Psychiatry*, **54**, 25–9.

Liu, Y., Stern, Y., Chun, M.R., Jacobs, D.M., Yau, P., & Goldman, J.E. (1997). Pathological correlates of extrapyramidal signs in Alzheimer's disease. *Annals of Neurology*, **41**, 368–74.

Lloyd, A.J. (1999). Comprehension of prosody in Parkinson's disease. *Cortex*, **35**, 389–402.

Lopez, O., Wisnieski, S.R., Becker, J.T., Boller, F., & DeKosky, S.T. (1997). Extrapyramidal signs in patients with probable Alzheimer disease. *Archives of Neurology*, **54**, 969–75.

Marder, K., Tang, M.X., Alfaro, B., et al. (1999). Risk of Alzheimer's disease in relatives of Parkinson's disease patients with and without dementia. *Neurology*, **52**, 719–24.

Marder, K., Tang, M.X., Cote, L., Stern, Y., & Mayeux, R. (1995). The frequency and associated risk factors for dementia in patients with Parkinson's disease. *Archives of Neurology*, **52**, 695–701.

Marttila, R.J., & Rinne, U.K. (1976). Dementia in Parkinson's disease. *Acta Neurologica Scandinavica*, **54**, 431–41.

Mattila, P.M., Rinne, J.O., Helenius, H., Dickson, D.W., & Roytta, M. (2000). Alpha-synuclein-immunoreactive cortical Lewy bodies are associated with cognitive impairment in Parkinson's disease. *Acta Neuropathologica*, **100**, 285–90.

Mayeux, R., Stern, Y., Rosen, J., & Leventhal, J. (1981). Depression, intellectual impairment, and Parkinson disease. *Neurology*, **31**, 645–50.

Mayeux, R., Stern, Y., Sano, M., Cote, L., & Williams, J.B.W. (1987). Clinical and biochemical correlates of bradyphrenia in Parkinson's disease. *Neurology*, **37**, 1130–4.

Merello, M., Sabe, L., Teson, A., et al. (1994). Extrapyramidalism in Alzheimer's disease: prevalence, psychiatric, and neuropsychological correlates. *Journal of Neurology, Neurosurgery and Psychiatry*, **57**, 1503–9.

Migliorelli, R., Teson, A., Sabe, L., Petracchi, M., Leiguarda, R., & Starkstein, S.E. (1995). Prevalence and correlates of dysthymia and major depression in Alzheimer's disease. *American Journal of Psychiatry*, **152**, 37–44.

Mindham, R.H.S. (1999). The place of dementia in Parkinson's disease: a methodologic saga. *Advances in Neurology*, **80**, 403–8.

Mitzutan, T., Aki, M., & Shiozawa, R. (1991). Clinicopathologic study of dementia in Parkinson's disease. *Dementia*, **2**, 229–36.

Mohr, E., Juncos, J., Cox, C., Litvan, I., Fedio, P., & Chase, T.N. (1990b). Selective deficits in cognition and memory in high-functioning Parkinsonian patients. *Journal of Neurology, Neurosurgery and Psychiatry*, **53**, 603–6.

Mohr, E., Litvan, I., Williams, J., Fedio, P., & Chase, T.N. (1990a). Selective deficits in Alzheimer and parkinsonian dementia: visuospatial function. *Canadian Journal of Neurological Sciences*, **17**, 292–7.

Mohr, E., Mendis, T., & Grimes, J.D. (1995). Late cognitive changes in Parkinson's disease with an emphasis on dementia. *Advances in Neurology*, **65**, 97–113.

Montgomery, P., Silverstein, P., & Wichmann, R. (1993). Spatial updating in Parkinson's disease. *Brain and Cognition*, **23**, 113–26.

Muller, U., Wachter, T., Barthel, H., Reuter, M., & von Cramon, D.Y. (2000). Striatal

[123I] beta-CIT SPECT and prefrontal cognitive functions in Parkinson's disease. *Journal of Neural Transmission*, **107**, 303–19.

Murray, A.M., Weihmueller, F.B., & Marshall, J.F. (1995). Damage to dopamine systems differs between Parkinson's disease and Alzheimer's disease with parkinsonism. *Annals of Neurology*, **37**, 300–12.

Nelson, H.E. (1976). A modified card sorting test sensitive to frontal lobe defects. *Cortex*, **12**, 313–24.

Owen, A.M., Doyon, J., Dagher, A., Sadikot, A., & Evans, A.C. (1998). Abnormal basal ganglia outflow in Parkinson's disease identified with PET: implications for higher cortical functions. *Brain*, **121**, 949–65.

Owen, A.M., Iddon, J.L., Hodges, J.R., Summers, B.A., & Robbins, T.W. (1997). Spatial and non-spatial working memory at different stages of Parkinson's disease. *Neuropsychologia*, **35**, 519–32.

Owen, A.M., Sahakian, B.J., Hodges, J.R., Summers, B.A., Polkey, C.E., & Robbins, T.W. (1995). Dopamine-dependent fronto-striatal planning deficits in early Parkinson's disease. *Neuropsychology*, **9**, 126–40.

Pascual-Leone, A., Grafman, J., & Clark, K. (1993). Procedural learning in Parkinson's disease and cerebellar degeneration. *Annals of Neurology*, **34**, 594–602.

Pate, D.S., & Margolin, D.I. (1994). Cognitive slowing in Parkinson's and Alzheimer's patients: distinguishing bradyphrenia from dementia. *Neurology*, **44**, 669–74.

Paulus, W., & Jellinger, K. (1991). The neuropathologic basis of different clinical subtypes of Parkinson's disease. *Journal of Neuropathology and Experimental Neurology*, **50**, 143–55.

Pell, J. (1996). On the receptive prosodic loss in Parkinson's disease. *Cortex*, **32**, 693–704.

Pillon, B., Deweer, B., Agid, Y., & Dubois, B. (1993). Explicit memory in Alzheimer's, Huntington's, and Parkinson's diseases. *Archives of Neurology*, **50**, 374–9.

Pillon, B., Dubois, B., Bonnet, A.M., et al. (1989). Cognitive slowing in Parkinson's disease fails to respond to levodopa treatment. *Neurology*, **39**, 762–8.

Pillon, B., Dubois, B., Lhermitte, F., & Agid, Y. (1986). Heterogeneity of cognitive impairment in progressive supranuclear palsy, Parkinson's disease, and Alzheimer's disease. *Neurology*, **36**, 1179–85.

Polich, J., Ehlers, C.L., Otis, S., Mandell, A.J., & Bloom, F.E. (1986). P300 latency reflects the degree of cognitive decline in dementing illness. *Electroencephalography and Clinical Neurophysiology*, **36**, 1179–85.

Portin, R., Laatu, S., Revonsuo, A., & Rinne, U.K. (2000). Impairment of semantic knowledge in Parkinson Disease. *Archives of Neurology*, **57**, 1338–43.

Rafal, R.D., Posner, M.J., Walker, J.A., & Friedrich, F.J. (1984). Cognition and the basal ganglia: separating mental and motor components of performance in Parkinson's disease. *Brain*, **107**, 1083–94.

Reid, W.G. (1992). The evolution of dementia in idiopathic Parkinson's disease: neuropsychological and clinical evidence in support of subtypes. *International Psychogeriatrics*, **4**, 147–60.

Richards, M., Stern, Y., & Mayeux, R. (1993). Subtle extrapyramidal signs can predict the development of dementia in elderly individuals. *Neurology*, **43**, 2184–8.

Rinne, J.O., Portin, R., Ruottinen, H., et al. (2000). Cognitive impairment and the brain dopaminergic system in Parkinson's disease. *Archives of Neurology*, **57**, 470–5.

Rinne, J.O., Rummukainen, J., Paljarvi, L., & Rinne, V.K. (1989). Dementia in Parkinson's disease is related to neuronal loss in the medial substantia nigra. *Annals of Neurology*, **26**, 47–50.

Robertson, C, & Empson, J. (1999). Slowed cognitive processing and high workload in Parkinson's disease. *Journal of Neurological Sciences*, **162**, 27–33.

Rogers, D., Lees, A.J., & Smith, E. (1987). Bradyphrenia in Parkinson's disease and psychomotor retardation in depressive illness: an experimental study. *Brain*, **110**, 761–6.

Roth, M., Huppert, F.A., Tym, E., & Mountjoy, C.Q. (1988). *CAMDEX. The Cambridge Examination for Mental Disorders of the Elderly*. Cambridge: Cambridge University Press.

Ruberg, M., & Agid, Y. (1988). Dementia in Parkinson's disease. In *Handbook of Psychopharmacology, Vol. 20, Psychopharmacology of aging nervous system*, ed. L.L. Iversen, S.D. Iversen & S.H. Snyder, pp. 157–206. New York: Plenum Press.

Sahakian, B.J., Morris, R.G., & Evenden, J.L. (1988). A comparative study of visuospatial memory and learning in Alzheimer type dementia and Parkinson's disease. *Brain*, **111**, 698–718.

Smith, M.C., Goldman, W.P., Janer, K.W., Baty, J.D., & Morris, J.C. (1998). Cognitive speed in nondemented Parkinson's disease. *Journal of the International Neuropsychological Society*, **4**, 584–92.

Sommer, M., Grafman, J., Clark, K., & Hallett, M. (1999). Learning in Parkinson's disease: eyeblink conditioning, declarative learning, and procedural learning. *Journal of Neurology, Neurosurgery and Psychiatry*, **67**, 27–34.

Starkstein, S.E., & Leiguarda, R. (1993). Neuropsychological correlates of brain atrophy in Parkinson's disease: a CT-scan study. *Movement Disorders*, **8**, 51–5.

Starkstein, S.E., Esteguy, M., Berthier, M.L., Garcia, H., & Leiguarda, R. (1989). Evoked potentials, reaction time and cognitive performance in on and off phases of Parkinson's disease. *Journal of Neurology, Neurosurgery and Psychiatry*, **52**, 338–40.

Starkstein, S.E., Leiguarda, R., Gershanik, L., & Berthier, M. (1987). Neuropsychological disturbances in hemi-parkinson's disease. *Neurology*, **37**, 1762–4.

Starkstein, S.E., Migliorelli, R., Manes, F., Teson, A., Petracca, G., & Chemerinski, E. (1995). The prevalence and clinical correlates of apathy and irritability in Alzheimer's disease. *European Journal of Neurology*, **2**, 1–7.

Starkstein, S.E., Sabe, L., Petracca, G., et al. (1996). Neuropsychological and psychiatric differences between Alzheimer's disease and Parkinson's disease with dementia. *Journal of Neurology, Neurosurgery and Psychiatry*, **61**, 381–7.

Starkstein, S.E., Vazquez, S., Petracca, G., Sabe, L., Merello, M., & Leiguarda, R. (1997). SPECT findings in Alzheimer's disease and Parkinson's disease with dementia. *European Journal of Neurology*, **4**, 231–6.

StClair, J.S., Borod, J.C., Sliwinski, M., Cote, L.J., & Stern, Y. (1998). Cognitive and affective functioning in Parkinson's disease patients with lateralized motor signs. *Journal of Clinical and Experimental Neuropsychology*, **20**, 320–7.

Stebbins, G.T., Gabrieli, J.D.E., Masciari, F., Monti, L., & Goetz, C.G. (1999). Delayed recognition memory in Parkinson's disease: a role for working memory? *Neuropsychologia*, **37**, 503–10.

Stern, Y., Mayeux, R., Sano, M., Hauser, W.A., & Bush, T. (1987). Predictors of disease course in patients with probable Alzheimer's disease. *Neurology*, **37**, 1649–53.

Stern, Y., Tang, M.X., Jacobs, D.M., et al. (1998). Prospective comparative study of the evolution of probable Alzheimer's disease and Parkinson's disease dementia. *Journal of the International Neuropsychological Society*, **4**, 279–84.

Tachibana, H., Aragane, K., Miyata, Y., & Sugita, M. (1997). Electrophysiological analysis of cognitive slowing in Parkinson's disease. *Journal of the Neurological Sciences*, **149**, 47–56.

Tison, F., Dartigues, J.F., Auriacombes, S., Letenneur, L., Boller, F., & Alperovitch, A. (1995). Dementia in Parkinson's disease: a population-based study in ambulatory and institutionalised individuals. *Neurology*, **45**, 705–8.

Tomer, R., Levin, B.E., & Weiner, W.J. (1993). Side of onset of motor symptoms influence cognition in Parkinson's disease. *Annals of Neurology*, **34**, 579–84.

Van der Borgh, T., Minoshima, S., Giordani, B., et al. (1997). Cerebral metabolic differences in Parkinson's and Alzheimer's diseases matched for dementia severity. *Journal of Nuclear Medicine*, **38**, 797–802.

Vermersch, P., Delacourte, A., Javoy-Agid, F., Hauw, J.J., & Agid, Y. (1993). Dementia in Parkinson's disease: biochemical evidence for cortical involvement using the immunodetection of abnormal Tau proteins. *Annals of Neurology*, **33**, 445–50.

Wermuth, L., Knudsen, L., & Boldsen, J. (1996). A study of cognitive functions in young Parkinsonian patients. *Acta Neurologica Scandinavica*, **93**, 21–4.

World Health Organization (1992). International classification of disease, tenth revision. The ICD–10 classification of mental and behavioral disorders. Clinical description and diagnostic guidelines. Geneva: World Health Organization.

Xuereb, J.H., Perry, E.K., & Candy, J.M. (1990). Parameters of cholinergic neurotransmission in the thalamus in Parkinson's disease and Alzheimer's disease. *Journal of Neurological Sciences*, **99**, 185–97.

Yoshimura, N., Yoshimura, I., & Asada, N. (1988). Juvenile Parkinson's disease with widespread Lewy bodies in the brain. *Acta Neuropathologica*, **77**, 213–18.

Zetusky, W.J., Jankovic, J., & Pirozzolo, F.J. (1985). The heterogeneity of Parkinson's disease: clinical and prognostic implications. *Neurology*, **35**, 522–6.

Zweig, R.M., Cardillo, J.E., Cohen, M., Giere, S., & Hedreen, J.C. (1993). The locus ceruleus and dementia in Parkinson's disease. *Neurology*, **43**, 986–91.

Chapter 5

American Psychiatric Association (1994). *Diagnostic and Statistical Manual of Mental Disorders*, 4th edn. Washington, DC: American Psychiatric Press.

Beck, A.T., Ward, C.M., & Mandelson, M. (1961). An inventory for measuring depression. *Archives of General Psychiatry*, **4**, 551–71.

Becker, G., Seufert, J., Bogdahn, U., Reichmann, H., & Reiners, K. (1995). Degeneration of substantia nigra in chronic Parkinson's disease visualized by transcranial duplex-sonography. *Neurology*, **45**, 182–4.

Becker, G., Struck, U., Bogdahn, U., & Becker, T. (1994). Echogenicity of the brainstem raphe in patients with major depression. *Psychiatry Research Neuroimaging*, **55**, 75–84.

Becker, T., Becker, G., Seufert, J., et al. (1997). Parkinson's disease and depression: evidence for an alteration of the basal limbic system detected by transcranial sonography. *Journal of Neurology, Neurosurgery and Psychiatry*, **63**, 590–6.

Bejjani, B.P., Damier, P., Arnulf, I., et al. (1999). Transient acute depression induced by high-frequency deep-brain stimulation. *New England Journal of Medicine*, **340**, 1476–80.

Boller, F., Marcie, P., Starkstein, S.E., & Traykov, L. (1998). Memory and depression in Parkinson's disease. *European Journal of Neurology*, **5**, 291–5.

Brown, R., & Jahanshahi, M. (1995). Depression in Parkinson's disease: a psychological viewpoint. *Advances in Neurology*, **65**, 61–84.

Brown, R.G., & MacCarthy, B. (1990). Psychiatric morbidity in patients with Parkinson's disease. *Psychological Medicine*, **20**, 77–87.

Brown, R.G., Jahanshahi, M., Quinn, N., & Marsden, C.D. (1990). Sexual function in patients with Parkinson's disease and their partners. *Journal of Neurology, Neurosurgery and Psychiatry*, **53**, 480–6.

Brown, R.G., MacCarthy, B., Gothan, A.M., Der, G.J., & Marsden, C.D. (1988). Depression and disability in Parkinson's disease: a follow-up of 132 cases. *Psychological Medicine*, **18**, 49–55.

Cantello, R., Aguggia, M., Gilli, M., et al. (1989). Major depression in Parkinson's disease and the mood response to intravenous methylphenidate: possible role of the "hedonic" dopamine synapse. *Journal of Neurology, Neurosurgery and Psychiatry*, **52**, 724–31.

Cantello, R., Gilli, M., Riccio, A., & Bergamasco, B. (1986). Mood changes associated with end-of-dose deterioration in Parkinson's disease: a controlled study. *Journal of Neurology, Neurosurgery and Psychiatry*, **49**, 1182–90.

Caroll, B.J., Feinberg, M., & Gredent, J.F. (1981). A specific laboratory test for the diagnosis of melancholia: standardization, validation and clinical utility. *Archives of General Psychiatry*, **38**, 15–22.

Cole, S.A., Woodard, J.L., Juncos, J.L., Kogos, J.L., Youngstrom, E.A., & Watts, R.L. (1996). Depression and disability in Parkinson's disease. *Journal of Neuropsychiatry and Clinical Neurosciences*, **8**, 20–5.

Davous, P., Auquier, P., Grignon, S., & Neukirch, H.C. (1995). A prospective study of depression in French patients with Parkinson's disease: the Depar study. *European Journal of Neurology*, **2**, 455–61.

Fahn, S., & Elton, E. (1987). Development Committee. Unified Parkinson's Disease Rating Scale, In *Recent Developments in Parkinson's Disease*, ed. S. Fahn, C.D. Marsden, M. Golstein & C.D. Calne. Florham Park, NJ: Macmillan.

Fetoni, V., Soliveri, P., Monza, D., Testa, D., & Girotti, F. (1999). Affective symptoms in multiple system atrophy and Parkinson's disease: response to levodopa therapy. *Journal of Neurology, Neurosurgery and Psychiatry*, **66**, 541–4.

Frochtengarten, M.L., Villares, J.G.B., & Maluf, E. (1987). Depressive symptoms and the dexamethasone suppression test in Parkinsonian patients. *Biological Psychiatry*, **22**, 386–9.

Gotham, A.M., Brown, R.G., & Marsden, C.D. (1986). Depression in Parkinson's disease: a quantitative and qualitative analysis. *Journal of Neurology, Neurosurgery and Psychiatry*, **49**, 381–9.

Hamilton, M. (1960). A rating scale for depression. *Journal of Neurology, Neurosurgery and Psychiatry*, **23**, 56–62.

Hantz, P., Caradoc-Davies, G., Caradoc-Davies, T., Weatherall, M., & Dixon, G. (1994). Depression in Parkinson's disease. *American Journal of Psychiatry*, **151**, 1010–14.

Hoehn, M.M., & Yahr, M.D. (1967). Parkinsonism: onset, progression and mortality. *Neurology*, **17**, 427–42.

Hoogendijk, W.J.G., Purba, J.S., Hofman, M.A., de Vos, R.A.I., Jansen, E.N.H., & Swaab, D.F. (1998a). Depression in Parkinson's disease is not accompanied by more corticotropin-releasing hormone expressing neurons in the hypothalamic paraventricular nucleus. *Biological Psychiatry*, **43**, 913–17.

Hoogendijk, W.J.G., Sommer, I.E.C., Tissingh, G., Deeg, D.J.H., & Wolters, E.Ch. (1998b). Depression in Parkinson's disease: the impact of symptom overlap on prevalence. *Psychosomatics*, **39**, 416–21.

Janet, P. (1924). Leçons sur les Maladies du Système Nerveux, 2nd edn. Paris: Delahaye.

Kostic, V.S., Sternic, N.C., & Bumbasirevic, L.B. (1990). Dexamethasone suppression test in patients with Parkinson's disease. *Movement Disorders*, **5**, 23–6.

Kuhn, W., Heye, N., Müller, T., et al. (1996a). The motor performance test series in Parkinson's disease is influenced by depression. *Journal of Neural Transmission*, **103**, 349–54.

Kuhn, W., Müller, T., Gerlach, M., et al. (1996b). Depression in Parkinson's disease: biogenic amines in CSF of "de novo" patients. *Journal of Neural Transmission*, **103**, 1441–5.

Kuopio, A.M., Marttila, R.J., Helenius, H., Toivonen, M., & Rinne, U.K. (2000). The quality of life in Parkinson's disease. *Movement Disorders*, **15**, 216–23.

Kuzis, G., Sabe, L., Tiberti, C., Leiguarda, R., & Starkstein, S.E. (1997). Cognitive functions in major depression and Parkinson's disease. *Archives of Neurology*, **54**, 982–6.

Leentjens, A.F., Verhe, F.R., Lousberg, R., Spitsbergen, H., & Wilmink, F.W. (2000). The validity of the Hamilton and Montgomery–Asberg depression rating scales as screening and diagnostic tools for depression in Parkinson's disease. *International Journal of Geriatric Psychiatry*, **15**, 644–9.

Levin, B.E., Llabre, M.M., & Weiner, W.J. (1988). Parkinson's disease and depression: psychomotor properties of the Beck Depression Inventory. *Journal of Neurology, Neurosurgery and Psychiatry*, **51**, 1401–4.

Liu, C.Y., Wang, S.J., Fuh, J.L., Lin, C.H., Yang, Y.Y., & Liu, H.C. (1997). The correlation of depression with functional activity in Parkinson's disease. *Journal of Neurology*, **244**, 493–8.

MacCarthy, B., & Brown, R. (1989). Psychosocial factors in Parkinson's disease. *British Journal of Clinical Psychology*, **28**, 41–52.

Maricle, R.A., Nutt, J.G., Valentine, R.J., & Carter, J.H. (1995). Dose–response relationship of levodopa with mood and anxiety in fluctuating Parkinson's disease: a double-blind, placebo-controlled study. *Neurology*, **45**, 1757–60.

Martinot, M.L.P., Bragulat, V., Artiges, E., et al. (2001). Decreased presynaptic dopamine function in the left caudate of depressed patients with affective flattening and psychomotor retardation. *American Journal of Psychiatry*, **158**, 314–16.

Mayberg, H.S., Brannan, S.K., Mahurin, R.K., et al. (1997). Cingulate function in depression: a potential predictor of treatment response. *Neuroreport*, **8**, 1057–61.

Mayberg, H.S., Starkstein, S.E., Sadzot, B., et al. (1990). Selective hypometabolism in the interior frontal lobe in depressed patients with Parkinson's disease. *Annals of Neurology*, **28**, 57–64.

Mayeux, R., Stern, Y., Cote, L., & Williams, J.B.W. (1984a). Altered serotonin metabolism in depressed patients with Parkinson's disease. *Neurology*, **34**, 642–6.

Mayeux, R., Williams, J.B.W., Stern, Y., & Cote, L. (1984b). Depression and Parkinson's disease. *Advances in Neurology*, **40**, 241–50.

Meara, J., Mitchelmore, E., & Hobson, P. (1999). Use of GDS–15 geriatric depression scale as a screening instrument for depressive symptomatology in patients with

Parkinson's disease and their carers in the community. *Age and Ageing*, **28**, 35–8.

Mellers, J.D., Quinn, N.P., & Ron, M.A. (1995). Psychotic and depressive symptoms in Parkinson's disease. A study of the growth hormone response to apomorphine. *British Journal of Psychiatry*, **167**, 522–6.

Menza, M.A., & Mark, M.H. (1993). Parkinson's disease and depression: the relationship to disability and personality. *Journal of Neuropsychiatry and Clinical Neurosciences*, **6**, 165–9.

Mindham, R.H.S. (1970). Psychiatric symptoms in parkinsonism. *Journal of Neurology, Neurosurgery and Psychiatry*, **33**, 188–91.

Montgomery, S.A., & Asberg, M. (1979). A new depression scale designed to be sensitive to change. *British Journal of Psychiatry*, **134**, 382–9.

Owen, A.M., Morris, R.G., Sahakian, B.J., Polkey, C.E., Robbins, T.W. (1996). Double dissociations of memory and executive functions in working memory tasks following frontal lobe excisions, temporal lobe excisions or amygdalo-hippocampectomy in man. *Brain*, **119**, 1597–615.

Pappert, E.J., Goetz, C.G., Niederman, F.G., Raman, R., & Leurgans, S. (1999). Hallucinations, sleep fragmentation, and altered dream phenomena in Parkinson's disease. *Movement Disorders*, **14**, 117–21.

Parkinson, J. (1817). *An Essay on the Shaking Palsy*. London: Sherwood, Neely & Jones.

Paulus, W. & Jellinger, K. (1991). The neuropathologic basis of different clinical subtypes of Parkinson's disease. *Journal of Neuropathology and Experimental Neurology*, **50**, 143–55.

Pilo, L., Ring, H., Quinn, N., & Trimble, M. (1996). Depression in multiple system atrophy and in idiopathic Parkinson's disease: a pilot comparative study. *Biological Psychiatry*, **39**, 803–7.

Raadsheer, F.C., Van Heerikhuize, J.J., Lucassen, P.J., Hoogendijk, W.J.G., Tilders, F.J.H., & Swaab, D.F. (1995). Corticotropin-releasing hormone mRNA levels in the paraventricular nucleus of patients with Alzheimer's disease and depression. *American Journal of Psychiatry*, **152**, 1372–6.

Richard, I.M., Justus, A.W., & Kurlan, R. (2001). Relationship between mood and motor fluctuations in Parkinson's disease. *Journal of Neuropsychiatry and Clinical Neurosciences*, **13**, 35–41.

Ring, H.A., Bench, C.J., Trimble, M.R., Brooks, K.J., Frackowiak, S.J., & Dolan, R.J. (1994). Depression in Parkinson's disease: a positron emission study. *British Journal of Psychiatry*, **165**, 333–9.

Robinson, R.G. (1998). *The Clinical Neuropsychiatry of Stroke*. Cambridge: Cambridge University Press.

Santamaría, J., Tolosa, E., & Valles, A. (1986). Parkinson's disease with depression: a possible subgroup of idiopathic parkinsonism. *Neurology*, **36**, 1130–3.

Schrag, A., Jahanshahi, M., & Quinn, N. (2000). What contributes to quality of life in patients with Parkinson's disease? *Journal of Neurology, Neurosurgery and Psychiatry*, **69**, 308–12.

Schrag, A., Jahanshahi, M., & Quinn, N. (2001). What contributes to depression in Parkinson's disease? *Psychological Medicine*, **31**, 65–73.

Serra-Mestres, J., & Ring, H.A. (1999). Vulnerability to emotionally negative stimuli in Parkinson's disease: an investigation using the emotional stroop task. *Neuropsychiatry, Neuropsychology, and Behavioral Neurology*, **12**, 52–7.

Singer, E. (1976). Sociopsychological factors influencing response to levodopa therapy for Parkinson's disease. *Archives of Physical Medicine and Rehabilitation*, **57**, 328–34.

Spitzer, R.L., William, J.B.W., & Gibbon, M. (1992). The structured clinical interview for DSM-III-R (SCID), I: history, rationale and description. *Archives of General Psychiatry*, **49**, 624–9.

Starkstein, S.E. (1999). Neurological models of depression. *Advances in Biological Psychiatry*, **19**, 123–35.

Starkstein, S.E., Berthier, M.L., Bolduc, P.L., Preziosi, T.J., & Robinson, R.G. (1989a). Depression in patients with "early" versus "late" onset of Parkinson's disease. *Neurology*, **39**, 1441–5.

Starkstein, S.E., Bolduc, P.L., Mayberg, H.S., Preziosi, T.J., & Robinson, R.G. (1990a). Cognitive impairments and depression in Parkinson's disease: a follow-up study. *Journal of Neurology, Neurosurgery and Psychiatry*, **53**, 597–602.

Starkstein, S.E., Bolduc, P.L., Preziosi, T.J., & Robinson, R.G. (1989b). Cognitive impairments in the different stages of Parkinson's disease. *Journal of Neuropsychiatry and Clinical Neurosciences*, **1**, 243–8.

Starkstein, S.E., Mayberg, H.S., Preziosi, T.J., & Robinson, R.G. (1992). A prospective longitudinal study of depression, cognitive decline, and physical impairments in patients with Parkinson's disease. *Journal of Neurology, Neurosurgery and Psychiatry*, **55**, 377–82.

Starkstein, S.E., Petracca, G., Chemerinski, E., et al. (1998). Depression in classic versus akinetic–rigid parkinson's disease. *Movement Disorders*, **13**, 29–33.

Starkstein, S.E., Preziosi, T.J., Berthier, M.L., Bolduc, P.L., Mayberg, H.S., & Robinson, R.G. (1989c). Depression and cognitive impairment in Parkinson's disease. *Brain*, **112**, 1141–53.

Starkstein, S.E., Preziosi, T.J., Bolduc, P.L., & Robinson, R.G. (1990b). Depression in Parkinson's disease. *Journal of Nervous and Mental Disease*, **178**, 37–41.

Starkstein, S.E., Preziosi, T.J., Forrester, A.W., & Robinson, R.G. (1990c). Specificity of affective and autonomic symptoms of depression in Parkinson's disease. *Journal of Neurology, Neurosurgery and Psychiatry*, **53**, 869–73.

Starkstein, S.E., Preziosi, T.J., & Price, T.R. (1991). Sleep disorders, pain and depression in Parkinson's disease. *European Neurology*, **31**, 352–5.

Tandberg, E., Larsen, J.P., Aarsland, D., & Cummings, J.L. (1996). The occurrence of depression in Parkinson's disease. *Archives of Neurology*, **53**, 175–9.

Tandberg, E., Larsen, J.P., Aarsland, D., Laake, K., & Cummings, J.L. (1997). Risk factors for depression in Parkinson disease. *Archives of Neurology*, **54**, 625–30.

Taylor, A.E., & Saint-Cyr, J.A. (1990). Depression in Parkinson's disease: reconciling physiological and psychological perspectives. *Journal of Neuropsychiatry and Clinical Neurosciences*, **2**, 92–8.

Tison, F., Barberger-Gateau, P., Dubroca, B., Henry, P., & Dartigues, J.F. (1997). Dependency in Parkinson's disease: a population-based survey in nondemented elderly subjects. *Movement Disorders*, **12**, 910–15.

Torack, R.M., & Morris, J.C. (1988). The association of ventral tegmental area histopathology with adult dementia. *Archives of Neurology*, **45**, 497–501.

Welsh, M., Hung, L., & Waters, C.H. (1997). Sexuality in women with Parkinson's disease. *Movement Disorders*, **12**, 923–7.

Wing, J.K., Cooper, E., & Sartorius, N. (1974). *Measurements and Classification of Psychiatric Symptoms*. Cambridge: Cambridge University Press.

World Health Organization (1992). The ICD-10 classification of mental and behavioral disorders. Clinical description and diagnostic guidelines. In *International Classification of Disease*, 10th revision. Geneva: World Health Organization.

Chapter 6

Aarsland, D., Larsen, J.P., Lim, N.G., et al. (1999). Range of neuropsychiatric disturbances in patients with Parkinson's disease. *Journal of Neurology, Neurosurgery and Psychiatry*, **67**, 492–6.

Bell, I.R., Schwartz, G.E., Amend, D., Peterson, J.M., Kaszniak, A.W., & Miller, C.S. (1994). Psychological characteristics and subjective intolerance for xenobiotic agents of normal young adults with trait shyness and defensiveness. A parkinsonian-like personality type? *Journal of Nervous and Mental Disease*, **182**, 367–74.

Booth, G. (1948). Psychodynamics in parkinsonism. *Psychosomatic Medicine*, **10**, 1–4.

Brooks, D.N., & McKinlay, W. (1983). Personality and behavioral change after severe blunt head injury: a relative's view. *Journal of Neurology, Neurosurgery and Psychiatry*, **46**, 336–44.

Camp, C.D. (1913). Paralysis agitans, multiple sclerosis and their treatment. In *Modern Treatment of Nervous and Mental Disease*, ed. W.A. White, S.E. Jelliffe & H. Kimpton, Vol. 2, pp. 651–7.

Cederbaum, J.M., & Aghajanian, G.K. (1977). Catecholamine receptors on locus coeruleus neurons: pharmacological characterisation. *European Journal of Pharmacology*, **44**, 375–85.

Charcot, J.M. (1875). *Leçons sur les Maladies du Système Nerveux*, 2nd edn, p. 179. Paris: Delahaye.

Charney, D.S., Grillon, C.M., & Brenner, D. (1998). The neurobiological basis of anxiety and fear: circuits, mechanisms, and neurochemical interactions. *The Neuroscientist*, **4**, 35–44.

Charney, D.S., Heninger, G.R., & Breier, A. (1984). Noradrenergic function in panic anxiety. Effects of yohimbine in healthy subjects and patients with agoraphobia and panic disorder. *Archives of General Psychiatry*, **41**, 751–63.

Costa, P.T., & McCrae, R.R. (1985). *The NEO Personality Inventory*. Odessa, FL: Psychological Assessment Resources.

Crow, T.J. (1972). A map of the rat mesencephalon for electrical self-stimulation. *Brain Research*, **36**, 265–73.

Dakof, G.A., & Mendelsohn, G.A. (1986). Parkinson's disease: the psychological aspects of a chronic illness. *Psychological Bulletin*, **99**, 375–87.

Eatough, V.M., Kempster, P.A., Stern, G.M., & Lees, A.J. (1990). Premorbid personality and idiopathic Parkinson's disease. *Advances in Neurology*, **53**, 335–7.

Fleminger, S. (1991). Left-sided Parkinson's disease is associated with greater anxiety and depression. *Psychological Medicine*, **21**, 629–38.

Folstein, M.F., Folstein, S.E., & McHugh, P.R. (1975). Mini-Mental State:a practical method for grading the cognitive state of patients for the clinician. *Journal of Psychiatric Research*, **12**, 189–98.

Fujii, C., Harada, S., Ohkoshi, N., Hayashi, A., & Yoshizawa, K. (2000). Cross-cultural traits for personality of patients with Parkinson's disease in Japan. *American Journal of Medical Genetics*, **96**, 1–3.

Glosser, G., Clark, C., Freundlich, B., Kliner-Krenzel, L., Flaherty, P., & Stern, M. (1995). A controlled investigation of current and premorbid personality: characteristics of Parkinson's disease patients. *Movement Disorders*, **10**, 201–6.

Gotham, A.M., Brown, R.G., & Marsden, C.D. (1986). Depression in Parkinson's disease: a quantitative and qualitative analysis. *Journal of Neurology, Neurosurgery and Psychiatry*, **49**, 381–9.

Hamilton, M. (1959). The assessment of anxiety states by rating. *British Journal of Medical Psychology*, **32**, 50–5.

Heberlein, I., Ludin, H.P., Scholz, J., & Vieregge, P. (1998). Personality, depression, and premorbid lifestyle in twin pairs discordant for Parkinson's disease. *Journal of Neurology, Neurosurgery and Psychiatry*, **64**, 262–6.

Hegeman-Richard, I.H., Szegethy, E., Lichter, D., Schiffer, R.B., & Kurlan, R. (1999). Parkinson's disease: a preliminary study of yohimbine challenge in patients with anxiety. *Clinical Neuropharmacology*, **22**, 172–5.

Hensler, J.G., Ferry, R.C., Labow, D.M., Kovachich, G.B., & Frazer, A. (1994). Quantitative autoradiography of the serotonin transporter to assess the distribution of serotonergic projections from the dorsal raphe nucleus. *Synapse*, **17**, 1–15.

Hubble, J.P., & Koller, W.C. (1995). The Parkinsonian personality. *Advances in Neurology*, **65**, 43–8.

Hubble, J.P., Ramachandran, V., Hassanein, R.E.S., Gray, C., & Koller, W.C. (1993). Personality and depression in Parkinson's disease. *Journal of Nervous and Mental Disease*, **181**, 657–62.

Iruela, L.M., Ibañez-Rojo, V., Palanca, J., & Caballero, L. (1992). Anxiety disorders and Parkinson's disease. *American Journal of Psychiatry*, **148**, 274.

Janet, P. (1924). *Leçons sur les Maladies du Système Nerveux*. Paris: Delahaye.

Labarca, C., Schwarz, J., Deshpande, P., et al. (2001). Point mutant mice with hypersensitive alpha 4 nicotinic receptors show dopaminergic deficits and increased anxiety. *Proceedings of the National Academy of Sciences*, **98**, 2786–91.

Maricle, R.A., Nutt, J.G., Valentine, R.J., & Carter, J.H. (1995). Dose–response relationship of levodopa with mood and anxiety in fluctuating Parkinson's disease: a double-blind, placebo-controlled study. *Neurology*, **45**, 1757–60.

Marin, R.S. (1991). Apathy: a neuropsychiatric syndrome. *Journal of Neuropsychiatry and Clinical Neurosciences*, **3**, 243–54.

Menza, M.A., & Mark, M.H. (1994). Parkinson's disease and depression: the relationship to disability and personality. *Journal of Neuropsychiatry and Clinical Neurosciences*, **61**, 165–9.

Menza, M.A., Forman, N.E., Goldstein, H.S., & Golbe, L.I. (1990). Parkinson's disease, personality, and dopamine. *Journal of Neuropsychiatry and Clinical Neurosciences*, **2**, 282–7.

Menza, M.A., Golbe, L.I., Cody, R.A., & Forman, N.E. (1993a). Dopamine-related personality traits in Parkinson's disease. *Neurology*, **43**, 505–8.

Menza, M.A., Mark, M.H., Burn, D.J., & Brooks, D.J. (1995). Personality correlates of [^{18}F] dopa striatal uptake: results of positron-emission tomography in Parkinson's disease. *Journal of Neuropsychiatry and Clinical Neurosciences*, **7**, 176–9.

Menza, M.A., Palermo, B., Di Paola, R., Sage, J.I., & Ricketts, M.H. (1999). Depression and anxiety in Parkinson's disease: possible effect of genetic variation in the serotonin transporter. *Journal of Geriatric Psychiatry and Neurology*, **12**, 49–52.

Menza, M.A., Roberston-Hoffman, D.E., & Bonapace, A.S. (1993b). Parkinson's disease and anxiety: comorbidity with depression. *Biological Psychiatry*, **34**, 465–70.

Mitscherlich, M. (1960). The psychic state of patients suffering from parkinsonism. In *Advances of Psychosomatic Medicine*, Vol. 1, pp. 317–24. Basel: Karger.

Poewe, W., Gerstenbrand, F., & Ransmayr, G. (1983). Premorbid personality of Parkinson patients. *Journal of Neural Transmission*, **19**, 215–24.

Poewe, W., Karamat, E., Kemmler, G.W., & Gerstenbrand, F. (1990). The premorbid personality of patients with Parkinson's disease: a comparative study with healthy controls and patients with essential tremor. *Advances in Neurology*, **53**, 339–42.

Rubin, A.J., Kurlan, R., Schiffer, R., Miller, C., & Shoulson, I. (1986). Atypical depression and Parkinson's disease. *Annals of Neurology*, **20**, 150.

Sands, I. (1942). The type of personality susceptible to Parkinson's disease. *Mount Sinai Journal of Medicine*, **9**, 792–4.

Schiffer, R.B., Kurlan, R., Rubin, A., & Boer, S. (1988). Evidence for atypical depression in Parkinson's disease. *American Journal of Psychiatry*, **145**, 1020–2.

Shiba, M., Bower, J.H., Maraganore, D.M., et al. (2000). Anxiety disorders and depressive disorders preceding Parkinson's Disease: a case-control study. *Movement Disorders*, **15**, 669–77.

Siemmers, E.R., Shekhar, A., Quaid, K., & Dickson, H. (1993). Anxiety and motor performance in Parkinson's disease. *Movement Disorders*, **8**, 501–6.

Speilberger, C.D. (1970). *Manual for the State-Trait Anxiety Inventory*. Palo Alto, CA: Consulting Psychologists' Press.

Starkstein, S.E. (2000). Apathy and withdrawal. *International Psychogeriatrics*, **12**, 135–8.

Starkstein, S.E., Mayberg, H.S., Preziosi, T.J., Andrezejewski, P., & Leiguarda, R. (1992). Reliability, validity and clinical correlates of apathy in Parkinson's disease. *Journal of Neuropsychiatry and Clinical Neurosciences*, **4**, 134–9.

Starkstein, S.E., Robinson, R.G., Leiguarda, R., & Preziosi, T.J. (1993b). Anxiety and depression in Parkinson's disease. *Behavioral Neurology*, **6**, 151–4.

Starkstein, S.E., Fedoroff, J.P., Price, T.R., Leiguarda, R., & Robinson, R.G. (1993a). Apathy following cerebrovascular lesions. *Stroke*, **24**, 1625–31.

Starkstein, S.E., Migliorelli, R., Manes, F., Teson, A., & Petracca, G. (1995). The prevalence and clinical correlates of apathy and irritability in Alzheimer's disease. *European Journal of Neurology*, **2**, 540–6.

Stein, M.B., Heuser, I.J., Juncos, J.L., & Uhde, T.W. (1990). Anxiety disorder in patients with Parkinson's disease. *American Journal of Psychiatry*, **147**, 217–20.

Toddes, C.J., & Lees, A.J. (1985). The pre-morbid personality of patients with Parkinson's disease. *Journal of Neurology, Neurosurgery and Psychiatry*, **48**, 97–100.

Vazquez, A., Jimenez-Jimenez, F.J., Garcia-Ruiz, P., & Garcia-Urra, D. (1993). "Panic attacks" in Parkinson's disease. A long-term complication of levodopa therapy. *Acta Neurologica Scandinavica*, **87**, 14–18.

Chapter 7

Aarsland, D., Larsen, J.P., Cummings, J.L., & Laake, K. (1999). Prevalence and clinical correlates of psychotic symptoms in Parkinson disease. A community-based study. *Archives of Neurology*, **56**, 595–601.

Absil, P., Das, S., & Balthazart, J. (1994). Effects of apomorphine on sexual behavior in male quail. *Pharmacology Biochemistry and Behavior*, **47**, 77–88.

Arnulf, I., Bonnet, A.M., Damier, P., et al. (2000). Hallucinations, REM sleep, and Parkinson's disease. A medical hypothesis. *Neurology*, **55**, 281–8.

Ball, B. (1882). De l'insanité dans la paralysie agitante. *Encéphale*, **2**, 22–32.

Banerjee, A.K., Flakai, P.G., & Savidge, M. (1989). Visual hallucinations in the elderly associated with the use of levodopa. *Postgraduate Medical Journal*, **65**, 358–61.

Brown, R.G., Marsden, C.D., Quinn, N., & Wyke, M.A. (1984). Alterations in cognitive performance and affect-arousal state during fluctuations in motor function in Parkinson's disease. *Journal of Neurology, Neurosurgery and Psychiatry*, **47**, 454–65.

Cooper, J.A., Sagar, H.J., & Sullivan, E.V. (1993). Short-term memory and temporal ordering in early Parkinson's disease: effects of disease chronicity and medication. *Neuropsychología*, **31**, 933–49.

Cummings, J.L. (1992). Neuropsychiatric complications of drug treatment of Parkinson's disease. In *Parkinson's Disease: Neurobehavioral Aspects*, ed. S.J. Huber & J.L. Cummings, pp. 313–27. New York: Oxford University Press.

De la Fuente-Fernandez, R., Nuñez, M.A., & Lopez, E. (1999). The apolipoprotein E4 allele increases the risk of drug-induced hallucinations in Parkinson's disease. *Clinical Neuropharmacology*, **22**, 226–30.

De Smet, Y., Ruberg, M., Serdaru, M., Dubois, B., Lhermitte, F., & Agid, Y. (1982). Confusion, dementia and anticholinergics in Parkinson's disease. *Journal of Neurology, Neurosurgery and Psychiatry*, **45**, 1161–4.

Diederich, N.J., Goetz, C.G., Raman, R., Pappert, E.J., Leurgans, S., & Piery, V. (1998). Poor visual discrimination and visual hallucinations in Parkinson's disease. *Clinical Neuropharmacology*, **21**, 289–95.

Dubois, B., Pillon, B., Llermitte, F., & Agid, Y. (1990). Cholinergic deficiency and frontal lobe dysfunction in Parkinson's disease. *Annals of Neurology*, **28**, 117–21.

Factor, S.A., Molho, E.S., & Brown, D.L. (1998). Acute delirium after withdrawal of amantadine in Parkinson's disease. *Neurology*, **50**, 1456–8.

Factor, S.A., Molho, E.S., Podskalny, G.D., & Brown, D. (1995). Parkinson's disease: drug-induced psychiatric states. *Advances in Neurology*, **65**, 115–38.

Fenelon, G., Mahieux, F., Huon, R., & Ziegler, M. (2000). Hallucinations in Parkinson's disease. Prevalence, phenomenology and risk factors. *Brain*, **123**, 733–45.

Fernandez, W., Stern, G., & Lees, A.J. (1992). Hallucinations and parkinsonian motor fluctuations. *Behavioral Neurology*, **5**, 83–6.

Friedberg, G., Zoldan, J., Weizman, A., & Melamed, E. (1998). Parkinson psychosis rating scale: a practical instrument for grading psychosis in Parkinson's disease. *Clinical Neuropharmacology*, **21**, 280–4.

Giladi, N., Treves, T.A., Paleacu, D., et al. (2000). Risk factor for dementia, depression and psychosis in long-standing Parkinson's disease. *Journal of Neural Transmission*, **107**, 59–71.

Giovannoni, G., O'Sullivan, J.D., Turner, K., Manson, A.J., & Lees, A.J.L. (2000).

Hedonistic homeostatic dysregulation in patients with Parkinson's disease on dopamine replacement therapies. *Journal of Neurology, Neurosurgery and Psychiatry*, **68**, 423–8.

Girotti, F., Carella, F., Grassi, M.D., Soliveri, P., Marano, R., & Caraceni, R. (1986). Motor and cognitive performances of parkinsonian patients in the on and off phases of the disease. *Journal of Neurology, Neurosurgery and Psychiatry*, **49**, 657–60.

Glantz, R.H., Bieliauskuas, L., & Paleologos, N. (1986). Behavioral indicators of hallucinosis in levodopa treated Parkinson's disease. *Advances in Neurology*, **45**, 417–20.

Goetz, C.G., & Stebbins, G.T. (1993). Risk factors for nursing home placement in advanced Parkinson's disease. *Neurology*, **43**, 2227–9.

Goetz, C.G., Burke, P.F., Leurgans, S., et al. (2001). Genetic variation analysis in Parkinson disease patients with and without hallucinations. Case-control study. *Archives of Neurology*, **58**, 209–13.

Goetz, C.G., Tanner, C.M., Gilly, G.W., et al. (1989). Development and progression of motor fluctuations and side effects in Parkinson's disease: comparison of Sinemet CR vs carbidopa/levodopa. *Neurology*, **39**, 63–6.

Goetz, C.G., Tanner, C.M., & Klawans, H.L. (1982). Pharmacology of hallucinations induced by long-term drug therapy. *American Journal of Psychiatry*, **139**, 494–8.

Graham, J.M., Grünewald, R.A., & Sagar, H.J. (1997). Hallucinosis in idiopathic Parkinson's disease. *Journal of Neurology, Neurosurgery and Psychiatry*, **63**, 434–40.

Growdon, J.H., Kieburtz, K., McDermott, M.P., Panisset, M., & Friedman, J.H. (1998). Levodopa improves motor function without impairing cognition in mild non-demented Parkinson's disease patients. Parkinson Study Group. *Neurology*, **50**, 1327–31.

Heaton, J.P. (2000). Apomorphine: an update of clinical trial results. *International Journal of Impotence Research*, **12**, S67–73.

Huber, S.J., Shulman, J.G., Paulson, G.W., et al. (1987). Fluctuations in plasma dopamine level impair memory in Parkinson's disease. *Neurology*, **37**, 1371–5.

Inzelberg, R., Kipervasser, S., & Koresyn, A.D. (1998). Auditory hallucinations in Parkinson's disease. *Journal of Neurology, Neurosurgery and Psychiatry*, **64**, 533–5.

Jankovic, J. (1985). Long-term study of pergolide in Parkinson's disease and progressive supranuclear palsy. *Neurology*, **35**, 296–9.

Jenkins, R.B., & Groh, R.H. (1970). Mental symptoms in parkinsonian patients treated with l-dopa. *Lancet*, **2**, 177–80.

Kieburtz, K., McDermott, M., Como, P., et al. (1994). The effect of deprenyl and tocopherol on cognitive performance in early untreated Parkinson's disease. *Neurology*, **44**, 1756–9.

Klawans, H.L. (1982). Behavioral alterations and the therapy of parkinsonism. *Clinical Neuropharmacology*, **5**, S29–37.

Kulisevsky, J., Avila, A., Barbano, M., Antonijoan, R., Berthier, M.L., & Gironell, A.

(1996). Acute effects of levodopa on neuropsychological performance in stable and fluctuating Parkinson's disease patients at different levodopa plasma levels. *Brain*, **119**, 2121–32.

Kulisevsky, J., Garcia-Sanchez, C., Berthier, M., et al. (2000). Chronic effects of dopaminergic replacement on cognitive function in Parkinson's Disease: a two-year follow-up study of previously untreated patients. *Movement Disorders*, **15**, 613–26.

Lange, K.W., Robbins, T.W., Marsden, C.D., James, M., Owen, A.M., & Paul, G.M. (1992). L-dopa withdrawal in Parkinson's disease selectively impairs cognitive performance in tests sensitive to frontal lobe dysfunction. *Psychopharmacology*, **107**, 394–404.

Lieberman, A., Leibowitz, M., Goppinathan, G., et al. (1985). The use of pergolide and lisuride, two experimental dopamine agonists, in patients with advanced Parkinson's disease. *American Journal of the Medical Sciences*, **290**, 102–6.

Makoff, A.J., Graham, J.M., Arranz, M.J., et al. (2000). Association study of dopamine receptor gene polymorphisms with drug-induced hallucinations in patients with idiopathic Parkinson's disease. *Pharmacogenetics*, **10**, 43–8.

Meco, G., Bonifati, V., Bedini, L., Bellatreccia, A., Vanacore, N., & Franzese, A. (1991). Relations between on–off phenomena and cognitive functions in Parkinson disease. *Italian Journal of Neurological Sciences*, **12**, 57–62.

Miyoshi, K., Ueki, A., & Nagano, O. (1996). Management of psychiatric symptoms of Parkinson's disease. *European Neurology*, **36**, 49–58.

Mohr, E., Fabbrini, G.G., Ruggieri, S., et al. (1987). Cognitive concomitants of dopamine system stimulation in parkinsonian patients. *Journal of Neurology, Neurosurgery and Psychiatry*, **60**, 1192–6.

Molina, J.A., Sainz-Artiga, M.J., Fraile, A., et al. (2000). Pathologic gambling in Parkinson's disease: a behavioral manifestation of pharmacologic treatment? *Movement Disorders*, **15**, 869–72.

Moskowitz, C., Moses, H., & Klawans, H.L. (1978). Levodopa-induced psychosis: a kindling phenomenon. *American Journal of Psychiatry*, **135**, 669–75.

Naimark, D., Jackson, E., Rockwell, E., & Jeste, D.V. (1996). Psychotic symptoms in Parkinson's disease patients with dementia. *Journal of the American Geriatrics Society*, **44**, 296–9.

Nausieda, P.A. (1985). Sinemet "abusers". *Clinical Neuropharmacology*, **8**, 318–27.

Nausieda, P.A., Weiner, W.J., & Klawans, H.L. (1982). Sleep disruption in the course of chronic levodopa therapy: an early feature of the levodopa psychosis. *Clinical Neuropharmacology*, **5**, 183–94.

Nissenbaum, H., Quinn, N.P., Brown, R.G., et al. (1990). Mood swings associated with the "on–off" phenomenon in Parkinson's disease. *Advances in Neurology*, **53**, 391–7.

O'Brien, C.P., DiGiacomo, J.N., Fahn, S., et al. (1971). Mental effects of high-dosage levodopa. *Archives of General Psychiatry*, **24**, 61–4.

Olson, E., Boeve, B.F., & Silber, M.H. (2000). Rapid eye movement sleep behavior disorder: demographic, clinical and laboratory findings in 93 cases. *Brain*, **123**, 331–9.

Overall, J.E., & Gorham, D.R. (1988). The brief psychiatric rating scale (BPRS): recent developments in ascertaining and scaling. *Psychopharmacology Bulletin*, **24**, 101–4.

Pappert, E.J., Goetz, C.G., Raman, R., Pass, M., & Leurgans, S. (1999). Hallucinations, sleep fragmentation, and altered dream phenomena in Parkinson's disease. *Movement Disorders*, **14**, 117–21.

Perry, E.K., & Perry, R.H. (1995). Acetylcholine and hallucinations: disease-related compared to drug-induced alterations in human consciousness. *Brain and Cognition*, **28**, 240–58.

Pillon, B., Dubois, B., Cusimano, G., Bonnet, A.M., Lhermitte, J., & Agid, Y. (1989). Does cognitive impairment in Parkinson's disease result from non-dopaminergic lesions? *Journal of Neurology, Neurosurgery and Psychiatry*, **52**, 201–6.

Pomerantz, S.M. (1992). Dopaminergic influences on male sexual behavior of rhesus monkeys: effects of dopamine agonists. *Pharmacology, Biochemistry and Behavior*, **41**, 511–17.

Przedsorski, S., Liard, A., & Hildebrand, J. (1992). Induction of mania by apomorphine in a depressed parkinsonian patient. *Movement Disorders*, **7**, 285–7.

Pullman, S.L., Watts, R.L., Juncos, J.L., et al. (1988). Dopaminergic effects on simple and choice reaction time performance in Parkinson's disease. *Neurology*, **38**, 249–54.

Quinn, N.P., Toone, B., Lang, A.E., et al. (1983). Dopa dose-dependent sexual deviation. *British Journal of Psychiatry*, **142**, 296–8.

Ruberg, M., Ploska, A., Javoy-Agid, F., & Agid, Y. (1982). Muscarinic binding and choline acetyltransferase activity in parkinsonian subjects with reference to dementia. *Brain Research*, **232**, 129–39.

Sanchez-Ramos, J.R., Ortoll, R., & Paulson, G.W. (1996). Visual hallucinations associated with Parkinson's disease. *Archives of Neurology*, **53**, 1265–8.

Shaw, K.M., Lees, A.J., & Stern, G.M. (1980). The impact of treatment with levodopa on Parkinson's disease. *Quarterly Journal of Medicine*, **49**, 283–93.

Svensson, T.H., Mathe, J.M., Andersson, J.L., Nomikos, G.G., Hilderbrand, B.E., & Marcus, M. (1995). Mode of action of a typical neuroleptic in relation of the phencyclidine model of schizophrenia: role of 5-HT2 receptor and alpha 1-adrenoceptor antagonism. *Journal of Clinical Psychopharmacology*, **15**, 11–18.

Tanner, C.M., Vogel, C., & Goetz, C.G. (1983). Hallucinations in Parkinson's disease: a population study. *Annals of Neurology*, **14**, 136.

Taylor, A.E., Saint-Cyr, J.A., & Lang, A.E. (1986). Frontal lobe dysfunction in Parkinson's disease: the cortical focus of neostriatal outflow. *Brain*, **109**, 845–83.

Teychenne, P.F., Bergstrund, D., Elton, R.L., et al. (1986). Bromocriptine: long-term low-dose therapy in Parkinson's disease. *Clinical Neuropharmacology*, **9**, 138–45.

The Parkinson Study Group (1990). Effect of Deprenyl on neuropsychological function in early untreated Parkinson's disease. *Annals of Neurology*, **28**, 336.

Timberlake, W.H., & Vance, M.A. (1978). Four-year treatment of patients with Parkinsonism using amantadine alone or with levodopa. *Annals of Neurology*, **3**, 119–28.

Vaamonde, J., Luquin, M.R., & Obeso, J.A. (1991). Subcutaneous lisuride infusion in Parkinson's disease. Response to chronic administration in 34 patients. *Brain*, **114**, 601–14.

van Spaencdonck, K.P.M., Berger, H.J.C., Horstink, M.W., Buytenhuijs, E.L., & Cools, A.R. (1993). Impaired cognitive shifting in Parkinsonian patients on anticholinergic therapy. *Neuropsychologia*, **31**, 407–11.

Chapter 8

Aarsland, D., Larsen, J.P., Karlsen, K., Lim, N.G., & Tandberg, E. (1999a). Mental symptoms in Parkinson's disease are important contributors to caregiver distress. *International Journal of Geriatric Psychiatry*, **14**, 866–74.

Aarsland, D., Larsen, J.P., Lim, N.G., & Tandberg, E. (1999b). Olanzapine for psychosis in patients with Parkinson's disease with and without dementia. *Journal of Neuropsychiatry and Clinical Neurosciences*, **11**, 392–4.

Allain, H., Pollak, P., & Neukirch, H.C. (1993). Symptomatic effect of selegiline in de novo parkinsonian patients: the French Selegiline Multicenter Trial. *Movement Disorders*, **8**, S36–40.

Andersen, J., Aabro, E., Gulmann, N., Hjelmested, A., & Pedersen, H.E. (1980). Anti-depressive treatment in Parkinson's disease: a controlled trial of the effect of nortriptyline in patients with Parkinson's disease treated with L-DOPA. *Acta Neurologica Scandinavica*, **62**, 210–19.

Anderson, K., Balldin, J., Gottfries, C.G., et al. (1987). A double-blind evaluation of electroconvulsive therapy in Parkinson's disease with "on–off" phenomena. *Acta Neurologica Scandinavica*, **76**, 191–9.

Auzou, P., Özsancak, A., Hannequin, D., Moore, N., & Augustin, P. (1996). Clozapine for the treatment of psychosis in Parkinson's disease: a review. *Acta Neurologica Scandinavica*, **94**, 329–36.

Balldin, J., Granerus, A., Linstedt, G., et al. (1981). Predictors for improvement after electroconvulsive therapy in parkinsonian patients with on–off symptoms. *Journal of Neural Transmission*, **52**, 199–211.

Barker, A.T., Freeston, I.L., Jalinous, R., & Jarratt, J.A. (1986). Clinical evaluation of conduction time measurements in central motor pathways using magnetic stimulation of the human brain. *Lancet*, **1**, 1325–6.

Bennett, J.P., Landow, E.R., & Schuh, L.A. (1993). Suppression of dyskinesias in advanced Parkinson's disease. II. Increasing daily clozapine doses suppresses dyskinesias and improves parkinsonism symptoms. *Neurology*, **43**, 1551–5.

Bonuccelli, U., Ceravolo, R., Salvetti, S., et al. (1997). Clozapine in Parkinson's disease tremor. Effects of acute and chronic administration. *Neurology*, **49**, 1587–90.

Bouchard, R.H., Purcher, E., & Vincent, P. (1989). Fluoxetine and extrapyramidal side effects. *American Journal of Psychiatry*, **146**, 1352–3.

Brown, R., & Jahanshahi, M. (1995). Depression in Parkinson's disease: a psychosocial viewpoint. *Advances in Neurology*, **65**, 61–84.

Caley, C.F., & Friedman, J.H. (1992). Does fluoxetine exacerbate Parkinson's disease? *Journal of Clinical Psychiatry*, **53**, 278–82.

Carter, J.H., Stewart, B.J., Archbold, P.G., et al. (1998). Living with a person who has Parkinson's disease: The spouse's perspective by stage of disease. *Movement Disorders*, **13**, 20–8.

Ceravolo, R., Nuti, A., Piccinni, A., et al. (2000). Paroxetine in Parkinson's disease: effects on motor and depressive symptoms. *Neurology*, **55**, 1216–18.

Coulter, D.M., & Pillans, P.I. (1995). Fluoxetine and extrapyramidal side effects. *American Journal of Psychiatry*, **152**, 122–5.

Dewey, R.B., & O'Suilleabhain, P.E. (2000). Treatment of drug-induced psychosis with quetiapine and clozapine in Parkinson's disease. *Neurology*, **55**, 1753–4.

Di Rocco, A., Rogers, J.D., Brown, R., Werner, P., & Bottiglieri, T. (2000). S-adenosyl-methionine improves depression in patients with Parkinson's disease in an Open-Label Clinical Trial. *Movement Disorders*, **15**, 1225–9.

Douyon, R., Serby, M., Klutchko, B., et al. (1989). ECT and Parkinson's disease revisited: a "naturalistic" study. *American Journal of Psychiatry*, **146**, 1451–5.

Eichorn, T.E., Brunt, B., & Oertel, A.H. (1996). Ondansetron treatment of L-dopa induced psychosis. *Neurology*, **47**, 1608–9.

Ellis, T., Cudkowicz, M.E., Sexton, P.M., & Growdon, J.H. (2000). Clozapine and Risperidone treatment of psychosis in Parkinson's disease. *Neurology*, **12**, 364–9.

Factor, S.A., & Brown, D. (1992). Clozapine prevents recurrence of psychosis in Parkinson's disease. *Movement Disorders*, **7**, 125–31.

Factor, S.A., & Friedman, J.H. (1997). The emerging role of clozapine in the treatment of movement disorders. *Movement Disorders*, **12**, 483–96.

Factor, S.A., Friedman, J.H., Lannon, M.C., Oakes, D., & Bourgeois, K. (2001). Clozapine for the treatment of drug-induced psychosis in Parkinson's disease: results of the 12 week open label extension in the PSYCLOPS trial. *Movement Disorders*, **16**, 135–9.

Factor, S.A., Molho, E.S., & Brown, D.L. (1995a). Combined clozapine and electrocon-vulsive therapy for treatment of drug-induced psychosis in Parkinson's disease. *Journal of Neuropsychiatry and Clinical Neurosciences*, **7**, 304–7.

Factor, S.A., Molho, E.S., Podskalny, G.D., & Brown, D. (1995b). Parkinson's disease: drug-induced psychiatric states. Advances in Neurology, **65**, 115–38.

Fava, M., Rosenbaum, J., Kolsky, A.R., et al. (1999). Open study of the catechol-0-methyltransferase inhibitor tolcapone in major depressive disorder. *Journal of Clinical Psychopharmacology*, **19**, 329–35.

Fernandez, H.H., Friedman J.H., Jacques, C., & Rosenfield M. (1999). Quetiapine for the treatment of drug-induced psychosis in Parkinson's disease. *Movement Disorders*, **14**, 484–7.

Fernandez, H.H., Lannon, M.C., Friedman, J.H., & Abbott, B.P. (2000). Clozapine replacement by quetiapine for the treatment of drug-induced psychosis in Parkinson's disease. *Movement Disorders*, **15**, 579–86.

Friedman, J.H. (1995). Managment of psychosis in Parkinson's disease. In *Therapy of Parkinson's Disease*, ed. W.C. Koller & G. Paulson, pp. 521–32. New York: Marcel Dekker.

Friedman, J.H. (1998). Olanzapine in the treatment of dopaminomimetic psychosis in patients with Parkinson's disease. *Neurology*, **50**, 1195–6.

Friedman, J.H., & Factor, S.A. (2000). Atypical antipsychotics in the treatment of drug-induced psychosis in Parkinson's disease. *Movement Disorders*, **15**, 201–11.

Friedman, J.H., & Lannon, M.C. (1989). Clozapine in the treatment of psychosis in Parkinson's disease. *Movement Disorders*, **39**, 1219–21.

Friedman, J.H., & Lannon, M.C. (1990). Clozapine treatment of tremor in Parkinson's disease. *Movement Disorders*, **5**, 225–9.

Friedman, J.H., Goldstein, S., & Jacques, C. (1998). Substituting clozapine for olanzapine in psychiatrically stable Parkinson's disease patients: results of an open label pilot study. *Clinical Neuropharmacology*, **21**, 285–8.

Garcia-Monco, J.C., Padierna, A., & Beldarrain, M.G. (1995). Selegiline, fluoxetine, and depression in Parkinson's disease. *Movement Disorders*, **10**, 352.

George, M.S., Wassermann, E.M., Kimbrell, T.A., et al. (1997). Mood improvement following daily left prefrontal repetitive transcranial magnetic stimulation in patients with depression: placebo-controlled crossover trial. *American Journal of Psychiatry*, **154**, 1752–6.

Goetz, C.G., Blasucci, L.M., Leurgans, S., & Pappert, E.J. (2000). Olanzapine and clozapine. Comparative effects on motor function in hallucinating PD patients. *Neurology*, **55**, 789–94.

Hargrave, R., & Ashford, J.W. (1992). Phenelzine treatment of depression in Parkinson's disease. *American Journal of Psychiatry*, **149**, 1751–2.

Hauser, A., & Zesiewicz, T.A. (1997). Sertraline for the treatment of depression in Parkinson's disease. *Movement Disorders*, **12**, 756–9.

Hegeman-Richard, I., Kurlan, R., & Parkinson Study Group (1997). A survey of antidepressant drug use in Parkinson's disease. *Neurology*, **49**, 1168–70.

Hurwitz, T.A., Calne, D.B., & Waterman, K. (1988). Treatment of dopaminomimetic psychosis in Parkinson's disease with electroconvulsive therapy. *Canadian Journal of*

Neurological Sciences, **15**, 32–4.

Indaco, A., & Carrieri, P.D. (1988). Amitriptyline in the treatment of headache in patients with Parkinson's disease. *Neurology*, 38, 1720–2.

Jansen Steur, E.N.H. (1993). Increase of parkinson disability after fluoxetine medication. *Neurology*, **43**, 211–13.

Jansen Steur, E.N.H. (1994). Clozapine in the treatment of tremor in Parkinson's disease. *Acta Neurologica Scandinavica*, **89**, 262–5.

Jansen Steur, E.N.H., & Ballering, L.A.P. (1999). Combined and selective monoamine oxidase inhibition in the treatment of depression in Parkinson's disease. *Advances in Neurology*, **80**, 505–8.

Jimenez-Jimenez, F.J., Tallón-Barranco, A., Ortí-Pareja, M., Zurdo, M., Porta, J., & Molina, J.A. (1998). Olanzapine can worsen parkinsonism. *Neurology*, **50**, 1183–4.

Jimenez-Jimenez, F.J., Tejeiro, J., Martinez-Junquera, G., Cabrera-Valdivia, F., Alarcon, J., & Garcia-Albea, E. (1994). Parkinsonism exacerbated by paroxetine. *Neurology*, **44**, 2406.

Juncos, J.L., Evatt, M.L., Jewart, R.D., et al. (2000). Long-term quetiapine for psychosis in Parkinson's disease in place of other antipsychotics. *Neurology*, **47**, 425.

Klaasen, T., Verhey, F.R.J., Sneijders, G.H.J.M., Rozendaal, N., Vet, H.V.W., & van Praag, H.M. (1995). Treatment of depression in Parkinson's disease: a meta-analysis. *Journal of Neuropsychiatry and Clinical Neurosciences*, **7**, 281–6.

Kurth, M.C., Adler, C.H., Hilaire, M.S., et al. (1997). Tolcapone improves motor function and reduces levodopa requirement in patients with Parkinson's disease experiencing motor fluctuations: a multicenter, double-blind, randomized, placebo-controlled trial. Tolcapone Fluctuator study group I. *Neurology*, **48**, 81–7.

Laitinen, L. (1969). Desipramine in the treatment of Parkinson's disease. *Acta Neurologica Scandinavica*, **45**, 109–13.

Leo, R.J. (1996). Movement disorders associated with the serotonin selective reuptake inhibitors. *Journal of Clinical Psychiatry*, **57**, 449–54.

Leopold, N.A. (2000). Risperidone treatment of Drug-Related Psychosis in patients with parkinsonism. *Movement Disorders*, **15**, 301–4.

Mally, J., & Stone, T.W. (1999). Therapeutic and "dose-dependent" effect of repetitive microelectroshock induced by transcranial magnetic stimulation in Parkinson's disease. *Journal of Neuroscience Research*, **57**, 935–40.

Manson, A.J., Schrag, A., & Lees, A.J. (2000). Olanzapine for levodopa induced dyskinesias. *Neurology*, **55**, 795–9.

Marty, M., Pouillart, P., & Scholl, S. (1990). Comparison of the 5-hydroxytryptamine$_3$ (serotonin) antagonist ondansetron (GR 38032F) with high-dose metoclopramide in the control of cisplatin-induced emesis. *New England Journal of Medicine*, **322**, 816–21.

Meara, R.J., Bhowmick, B.K., & Hobson, J.P. (1996). An open uncontrolled study of the use of sertraline in the treatment of depression in Parkinson's disease. *Journal of Serotonin Research*, **4**, 243–9.

Meco, G., Alessandri, A., Giustini, P., & Bonifati, V. (1997). Risperidone in levodopa-induced psychosis in Parkinson's disease: an open-label, long-term study. *Movement Disorders*, **12**, 610–11.

Moellentine, C., Rummans, T., Ahlskog, J.E., et al. (1998). Effectiveness of ECT in patients with parkinsonism. *Journal of Neuropsychiatry and Clinical Neurosciences*, **10**, 187–93.

Mohr, E., Mendis, T., Hildebrand, K., & De Deyn, P.P. (2000). Risperidone in the treatment of Dopamine-Induced Psychosis in Parkinson's Disease: an open pilot trial. *Movement Disorders*, **15**, 1230–7.

Montastruc, J.L., Fabre, N., Blin, O., et al. (1994). Does fluoxetine aggravate Parkinson's disease? A pilot prospective trial. *Movement Disorders*, **9**, 99.

Musser, W.S., & Mayada, A. (1996). Clozapine as a treatment for psychosis in Parkinson's disease: a review. *Journal of Neuropsychiatry and Clinical Neurosciences*, **8**, 1–9.

Pakkenberg, H., & Pakkenberg, B. (1986). Clozapine in the treatment of tremor. *Acta Neurologica Scandinavica*, **73**, 295–7.

Parsa, M.A., & Bastani, B. (1998). Quetiapine (Seroquel) in the treatment of psychosis in patients with Parkinson's disease. *Journal of Neuropsychiatry and Clinical Neurosciences*, **10**, 216–19.

Pinter, M.M., & Helscher, R.J. (1993). Therapeutic effect of clozapine in psychotic decompensation in idiopathic Parkinson's disease. *Journal of Neural Transmission*, **5**, 135–46.

Rasmussen, K.G., & Abrams, R. (1992). The role of electroconvulsive therapy in Parkinson's disease. In *Parkinson's Disease: Neurobehavioral Aspects*, ed. S.J. Huber & J.L. Cummings, pp. 255–70. New York: Oxford University Press.

Richard, I., Kurlan, R., & Tanner, C. (1997). Serotonin syndrome and combined use of deprenyl and an antidepressant in Parkinson's disease: Parkinson Study Group. *Neurology*, **48**, 1070–7.

Roberts, H.E., Dean, R.C., & Stoudemire, A. (1989). Clozapine treatment of psychosis in Parkinson's disease. *Journal of Neuropsychiatry and Clinical Neurosciences*, **1**, 190–2.

Ruggieri, S., Pandis, M.F., Bonamartini, A., Vacca, L., & Stocchi, F. (1997). Low dose of clozapine in the treatment of dopaminergic psychosis in Parkinson's disease. *Clinical Neuropharmacology*, **20**, 204–9.

Singer, E. (1973). Social costs of Parkinson's disease. *Journal of Chronic Disease*, **26**, 243–54.

Starkstein, S.E., Mayberg, H.S., Preziosi, T.J., & Robinson, R.G. (1992). A prospective longitudinal study of depression, cognitive decline, and physical impairments in patients with Parkinson's disease. *Journal of Neurology, Neurosurgery and Psychiatry*, **55**, 377–82.

Sternbach, H. (1991). The serotonin syndrome. *American Journal of Psychiatry*, **148**, 705–13.

Strang, R.R. (1965). Imipramine in treatment of parkinsonism: a double-blind placebo study. *British Medical Journal*, **2**, 33–4.

Targum, S.D., & Abbott, J.L. (2000). Efficacy of quetiapine in Parkinson's patients with psychosis. *Journal of Clinical Psychopharmacology*, **20**, 54–60.

Tesei, S., Antonini, A., Canesi, M., Zecchinelli, A., Mariani, C.B., & Pezzoli, G. (2000). Tolerability of paroxetine in Parkinson's disease: a prospective study. *Movement Disorders*, **15**, 986–9.

The French Clozapine Parkinson Study Group (1999). Clozapine in drug-induced psychosis in Parkinson's disease. *Lancet*, **353**, 2041–2.

The Parkinson Study Group (1999). Low-dose clozapine for the treatment of drug-induced psychosis in Parkinson's disease. *New England Journal of Medicine*, **340**, 757–63.

Tom, T. & Cummings, J.L. (1998). Depression in Parkinson's disease. Pharmacological characteristics and treatment. *Drugs and Aging*, **12**, 55–74.

Trosch, R.M., Friedman, J.H., Lannon, M.C., et al. (1998). Clozapine use in Parkinson's disease: a retrospective analysis of a large multicentered clinical experience. *Movement Disorders*, **13**, 377–82.

Valldeoriola, F., Nobbe, F.A., & Tolosa, E. (1997). Treatment of behavioral disturbances in Parkinson's disease. *Journal of Neural Transmission*, **51**, 175–204.

Wagner, M.L., Pharm, D., Defilippi, J.L., Menza, M.A., & Sage, J.I. (1996). Clozapine for the treatment of psychosis in Parkinson's disease: chart review of 49 patients. *Journal of Neuropsychiatry and Clinical Neurosciences*, **8**, 276–80.

Waters, C.H. (1994). Fluoxetine and selegiline: lack of significant interaction. *Canadian Journal of Neurological Sciences*, **21**, 259–61.

Wolters, E.Ch. (1999). Dopaminomimetic psychosis in parkinson's disease patients. Diagnosis and treatment. *Neurology*, **52**, S10–S13.

Wolters, E.Ch., Jansen, E.N.H., Tuynman-Qua, H.G., & Bergmans, P.L.M. (1996). Olanzapine in the treatment of dopaminomimetic psychosis in patients with Parkinson's disease. *Neurology*, **47**, 1085–7.

Workman, R.H., Orengo, C.A., Bakey, A.A., Molinari, V.A., & Kunik, M.E. (1997). The use of risperidone for psychosis and agitation in demented patients with Parkinson's disease. *Journal of Neuropsychiatry and Clinical Neurosciences*, **9**, 594–7.

Zoldan, J., Friedberg, G., Livneh, M., & Melamed, E. (1995). Psychosis in advanced Parkinson's disease: treatment with ondansetron, a 5-HT3 receptor antagonist. *Neurology*, **45**, 1305–8.

Appendix

Friedberg, G., Zoldan, J., Weizman, A., & Melamed, E. (1998). Parkinson Psychosis Rating Scale: a practical instrument for grading psychosis in Parkinson's disease. *Clinical Neuropharmacology*, **21**, 280–4.

Goetz, C.G., Stebbins, G., Shale, H.M., et al. (1994). Utility of one objective dyskinesia rating scale for PD. Inter and intrarater reliability assessment. *Movement Disorders*, **9**, 390–4.

Lang, A.E. (1990). Clinical rating scale and videotapes analysis. In *Therapy of Parkinson Disease*, ed. W.C. Koller & G. Paulsen, pp. 3–30. New York: Marcel Dekker.

Langston, J.W., Widner, H., Goetz, C.G., et al. (1992). Core Assessment Program for Intracerebral Transplantation (CAPIT). *Movement Disorders*, **7**, 2–13.

Nouzeilles, M.I., & Merello, M. (1997). Correlation between results of motor section of UPDRS and Webster scale. *Movement Disorders*, **12**, 613.

Schrag, A., Jahanshahi, M., & Quinn, N. (2000). How does Parkinson's disease affect quality of life? A comparison with quality of life in the general population. *Movement Disorders*, **15**, 1112–18.

Starkstein, S.E., Mayberg, H.S., Preziosi, T.J., Andrezejewski, P., Leiguarda, R., & Robinson, R.G. (1995). Reliability, validity, and clinical correlates of apathy in Parkinson's disease. *Journal of Neuropsychiatry and Clinical Neurosciences*, **4**, 134–9.

Webster, D. (1968). Critical analysis of the disability in Parkinson's disease. *Medical Treatment*, **5**, 257–82.

Index

Printed in the United States
By Bookmasters